Disclaimer

I0103871

Welcome to Absurdistan

Absurdistan may be imaginary, but that hasn't prevented its narrators from sneaking in through the cracks in our world, smuggling these pages into the other side of reality, like some sort of literary contraband. Before we get started, though, let's take a moment for a brief but needed word of caution.

No Replacement for Professional Guidance

This book is intended for general information, entertainment and educational purposes only. It is not intended to be a substitute for professional, medical, psychological, or mental health diagnosis, treatment, or advice. If you have any concerns about your physical or mental health, please consult a qualified healthcare provider or a licensed mental health professional. The writer is not a doctor or licensed clinician, and the information in this is never a substitute for appropriate care.

Limitation of Liability and User Responsibility

The author and the publisher are herewith absolved and rid of all liability by reader. Readers are advised to use their own judgment in making decisions in any areas pertaining to their life, health, and financial wellbeing. Whatever you decide to be inspired by is ultimately your prerogative, so if you do swing wildly through Absurdistan, be sure to do so with a sprinkling of common sense and self-awareness.

Continuing means you've read and understood this disclaimer, accepting that the information isn't professional advice. Consider it a courtesy signal that the absurd universe has begun. Let's step into the story, contraband and all, enjoy the ride!

Chapter 1: Introduction

When life backs you into a bathroom stall, wipe your tears, fix your smile, and step out like you own the place. Half the magic is just daring to show up.

I never pictured myself writing a self-help book., and certainly not one about mental health. And yet, here I am, presenting these pages Half Crazy, Fully Human. It sums up the paradox of how we can feel borderline overwhelmed, "half crazy", and yet remain, at the same time, fully capable of resilience and growth. For years, I embodied that paradox firsthand: the person crying in a restroom stall at office parties, hastily wiping away tears, then bursting out with jokes and a theatrical smile as though nothing was wrong. Humor was like my armor, a dress-up filter that duped everyone (and occasionally me) into thinking I was okay. But at some point, that armor faltered. Looking through the cracks, I discovered what was gently assertive: hope. As we are on this path, do not forget that experiencing professional help is courageous. Chapter 1: Introduction When life puts you in a bathroom stall, wipe your tears, put on your smile, and step out like you own the place. And half the magic is simply having the courage to show up. While I'm not a licensed professional, this book merges personal narratives with scientific references. However, proper mental health advice from qualified practitioners is best tailored to the individual. Please use these pages with your therapy, not instead of it. If you ever feel too low or stressed to handle, remember that talking to a mental health professional, a crisis line, or someone you trust in your community is a sign of strength and self-care.

This book tells the story of how I put together the pieces of my broken mind, learned to laugh again (really laugh), and faced the storm of feelings that had once threatened to destroy me. If any of this sounds like something you've experienced, nighttime cycles of overthinking hidden by pleasantries during the day, know that you are not alone. A lot of us deal with worry, depression, and self-doubt in our heads, which aren't always welcome. From 9 to 5, we act strong, but we break down when the doors are closed. However, it can be courageous to admit that life is hard and look for funny things along the way. If you're going through mental shivers, I've been there, found tools (and the occasional 2 a.m. dance party in my kitchen), and come away with stories that might connect with you. You're not alone in this journey.

I'm not going to say that laughing makes everything better. Fundamental problems with mental health go deep, and they should get professional help when they happen. Researchers have found that humor can help us deal with our fears more acceptably (Martin, 2010; Mayo Clinic, 2023.). You can expect personal stories and references to scientifically sound ideas in the following parts. Think of it like a roller coaster ride: there will be bumps, drops, screams, and hopefully some fantastic views by the end.

A Glimpse at the Path Ahead

You and I start this relationship here in Chapter One. We get to know each other beyond the book cover. Right? Then, together, we move on to Chapter 2, exploring the notion that "ignorance is bliss," at least in some cases. We will look at whether avoiding too much bad news on purpose can be good for mental health (Sweeny et al., 2010) and when that avoidance turns into harmful denial. Chapter 3 expands on this theme by showing how changing your point of view, like pretending to be an alien anthropologist, can make everyday stresses seem silly (Martin, 2010). When you realize you're about to lose it over a few "unread emails," they might seem funny or at least less scary.

From there, Chapter 4 explores the question of whether "money can't buy happiness," presenting research suggesting that while money may reduce financial insecurity, long-term well-being generally comes from relationships, meaning, and growth (Diener et al., 2018; Kahneman & Deaton, 2010; Killingsworth, 2023). Chapter 5 turns inward to the inner tempest of an anxious or overthinking mind and how we unravel chaos and restore calm. Chapter 6 offers the approach, "no pain, no gain" (Meichenbaum, 1988), leading us to a middle ground in Reich and Zautra (2010) where a "limited amount" of struggle helps us to survive and flourish, yet too much adversity can crush.

Then, Chapter 7 cautions us against judging a book by its cover as it illustrates how appearances deceive us. Chapter 8 deals with depression, how it is separate from anxiety, how numbness can muffle tears, and how small acts lead to momentum. Chapter 9 embraces the idea of "failing spectacularly" or that mistakes, when owned honestly, give much greater wisdom than instantaneous wins (Eskreis-Winkler & Fishbach, 2019). Chapter 10 examines the power of humor in relationships, while Chapter 11 weighs caution against opportunity in "better safe than sorry."

By Chapter 12, we've talked about how our phone-clutching reaction stops us from being bored and the creative ideas that can come from it (Eastwood et al., 2012). Finally, Chapter 13 brings all these ideas together by thinking about how to keep growing, how laughter helps us stay strong, and why none of us are "broken" or "fixed."

Taking Our First Steps

So, whether you're reading these lines out of mild interest or desperately need help, I hope you find something that speaks to you. Heartbreak, anxiety, self-doubt, and even existential problems about our worth happen to everyone at some point in their lives. In exploring these chapters, you'll see that humor can be a quiet ally and that messy minds can still hold enormous promise. Let's see how far a blend of introspection, levity, and sincere willingness to keep going can take us.

Remember, growth is always possible; this book is a testament to that.

If you find yourself still wiping tears in a bathroom stall, realize that stepping out, nervous grin and all, could be half the magic. The rest is discovering, as we walk on, that fragile moments can birth hope and that a small, wry smile might be enough to lighten even the heaviest load. We'll head next into why "ignorance can be bliss," at least occasionally, before questioning how perspective, finances, relationships, failure, and boredom intertwine in a tapestry that calls us to keep growing. And yes, Volume 2 will eventually tackle the family influences and other themes that needed a dedicated space.

Welcome to Half Crazy, Fully Human. For however long you choose to stay. Let's begin.

Chapter 2: Up to a Point, Ignorance Is Bliss

Blissful ignorance can feel like a hammock on a sunny afternoon, comfortable while it lasts, but eventually the bugs show up and reality wants you back.

On a dinner party in a warm suburban living room, the conversation shifts from small talk about the weather to the state of the world. By dessert, an elegantly constructed chocolate torte, two voices dominate the conversation: Alice's and Bob's. Alice fires off a barrage of alarming statistics she has amassed over the past week: political turmoil in half a dozen countries, new pandemic risks, signs of a looming recession. Her anxious tone suggests she has been mentally scripting doomsday scenarios for days now.

Bob listens quietly and shrugs. He smiles and admits that he hasn't seen the news in weeks. Instead, he spends his days tending to his flowerbeds and watching reruns of old sitcoms. A hush falls over the table. Alice regards him with exasperation and disbelief, she calls him irresponsible for refusing to stay updated on global calamities, while Bob studies his slice of torte with undisturbed calm, as though he's stepped away from an invisible tempest. The question is: Is Bob's calm detachment helpful, or is it an illusion that will catch up with him when reality knocks?

People have debated the pros and cons of "not knowing" for centuries. The saying "ignorance is bliss" applies to personal, social, and even transcendental life. On the one hand, an excess of alarming information can swamp us. On the other, living in a state of permanent blind spots may lead to reckless complacency. We will explore the origins of this proverb and how it applies in real life throughout this chapter, delving into psychological research on when and why people avoid information, the consequences of excessive knowledge or persistent ignorance, and ways to find a middle ground that protects mental health without leaving us vulnerable to real dangers. Along the way, we'll return to Alice and Bob, two radically different mindsets at the same table, to see what their story reveals about human nature.

Lure and Limits of Selective ignorance

Ignorance as bliss is appealing in our time due to constant news and social media feeds, which researchers call "information overload" (Sweeny et al., 2010). Phone alerts, 24-hour news channels, podcasts, and headlines invade our screens, making it difficult to escape. Unfortunately, much of what we see is dark: natural disasters, economic uncertainties, and tense political standoffs. In a world where problems seem global and immediate, many people experience anxiety or hopelessness. Ignorance becomes a sanctuary, a respite from psychological overload.

When Bob says he'd rather be in his garden or binging comedy reruns than following every new crisis, he expresses a point of view that's been on the rise. Studies from the first months of the 2020 pandemic showed that people high in analytic thinking who consumed a lot of daily COVID-19 news saw steeper declines in life satisfaction than those who paid less attention to the crisis (Kanazawa & Li, 2018). The latter group, much like Bob, seemed to fare better, at least in the short term. Critics label this kind of selective ignorance as a form of neglect, yet its advocates argue that humans are not designed, psychologically or biologically, to shoulder global woes constantly. Endless vigilance might promise a feeling of control, but paradoxically, it can corrode mental health.

There is a certain logic behind "what you don't know can't hurt you," at least for a while. People generally prefer not to confront unsettling information if they doubt, they can do much to change it. Some individuals choose not to view genetic test results if no cure exists for a potentially inherited condition, or dodge checking their bank account if they suspect the balance is low (Sweeny et al., 2010). This preference for ignorance can bring short-lived relief by postponing the anxiety that knowledge might ignite. As a coping mechanism, ignorance is a breather: if you never notice the coming storm clouds, you won't fret about the rain. Would you?

The Wisdom of Knowing You Know Nothing

However soothing the approach sounds, it overlooks that problems do not vanish the moment we stop looking at them. In the dinner party analogy, Bob's composure might be severely tested if a major emergency lies ahead, like a serious hurricane heading for the region. If he tunes out all news, he might neglect to stock up on supplies or evacuate in time. Less drastically, ignoring a strange rattling noise in your car on the grounds that you'd "rather not deal with it" can spare you today's hassle but might lead to a car breakdown tomorrow. Likewise, skipping doctor visits to avoid worrying about test results could cause you to miss something treatable in its early stages.

The proverb "ignorance is bliss" has roots in a poetic line by Thomas Gray in the 18th century: "Where ignorance is bliss, 'tis folly to be wise." It was originally a reflection on the innocence of youth, how children, oblivious to adult realities, can freely chase fun. This poetic notion suggests that knowledge carries burdens. Indeed, as kids, we long to be "grown-ups," only to discover that adulthood brings a host of responsibilities and sobering truths we never anticipated. If everyone collectively opted for childlike obliviousness, society would stall. Painful facts drive scientific innovation, medical breakthroughs, and social progress. So, while Gray's line may capture the comfort of fleeting unawareness, genuine growth demands we confront difficulties.

That tension between not knowing and actively engaging becomes sharper when we consider moral obligations. Willful blindness, deliberately ignoring wrongdoing or urgent crises, can be not just a personal flaw but an ethical one. History holds plenty of examples of governments or large groups dismissing disasters until it was too late. There is a tragic or comic vision of an ostrich burying its head in the sand: a convenient metaphor for refusing to see a mounting problem, snagging a moment of illusory peace while the horizon darkens.

Alice, at the dinner party, presents the opposite extreme from Bob. She's inundated with every grim detail. Her anxiety spills into casual gatherings, overshadowing the gentle murmur of conversation. She may be ready for worst-case scenarios, fully stocked on necessities, deeply informed on politics and scientific data fueling the headlines, but that constant sense of urgency weighs heavily on her. If she cannot compartmentalize, she might become perpetually tense, sleepless, and depleted, knowing she cannot single-handedly fix all crises nor flip off her hyper-vigilance. From a mental health angle, oversaturation with negative stories can lead to catastrophizing and chronic stress (Brooks et al., 2020). The term "doomscrolling" has emerged to describe the compulsion to keep reading bad news, fueling a cycle of alarm.

Alice and Bod Extremes

Neither extreme, Bob's blissful ignorance nor Alice's oversaturation, is particularly healthy. Bob's self-imposed detachment leaves him vulnerable to real threats and personal oversights. Alice's on-edge vigilance erodes her ability to savor life's joys. Their experiences caricature the two poles: one with no lens on current affairs, the other drowning in a nonstop feed of grim updates. On a broader social scale, entire communities can slip into one camp or the other. Some pride themselves on being incessant news hounds, always up to date but teetering on the brink of anxiety. Others adopt a communal silence, refusing to "rock the boat with negativity," sustaining a fragile tranquility that shatters at the first sign of real trouble.

From a psychological standpoint, this phenomenon is called information avoidance (Sweeny et al., 2010) and can be understood through stress-and-coping models proposed by Lazarus and Folkman (1984). Avoiding stressful information does lower emotional distress in the short run, but if the stressor is genuine and solvable, that approach typically fails over time, leading to bigger problems. Bob's style of ignorance might be the milder type: turning off the news after 7 p.m. so it won't disturb his sleep. That could be wise self-preservation. But if he never checks the news at all, always playing catch-up with urgent events, he drifts from a coping strategy into a damaging habit.

Many people attempt a middle path. They opt for a "less is more" media approach, maybe skimming key headlines once a day from reputable outlets, reading more deeply only as needed, then deliberately unplugging to focus on personal goals or rest. Some call this intentional ignorance, not burying your head in the sand but choosing when and how to immerse yourself in weighty content. A friend of mine, Tanya, instituted "News-Free Mondays," using that one weekly day to read no news, limiting social media, and concentrating on journaling or creative hobbies. She discovered that skipping just that single day of updates preserved her sanity, and she could still remain reasonably informed the other six days.

In personal relationships, ignorance can also masquerade as a peacekeeper. Sometimes, people say they'd rather not know every gripe or bit of gossip, hoping to avoid unnecessary friction. While such micro-ignorance can avert petty quarrels, they, too, have boundaries. If a friend harbors a serious grievance or a partner quietly wrestles with a crisis, not knowing can result in missed connections or lost chances to help.

A deeper historical or cultural view shows that "ignorance is bliss" predates the modern world. Thomas Gray's poem and Voltaire's satirical Candide revolve around naive optimism shattered by reality's harshness. Voltaire's Pangloss insists all is for the best in "this best of all possible worlds," providing comedic relief in fiction but reading as negligence in real life. Some ancient philosophical traditions counseled limiting knowledge to maintain inner peace, yet they, too, recognized that ignoring the fundamental nature of the world would not breed genuine wisdom.

Bob and Alice in the aftermath of this dinner confrontation, Bob might head home untroubled, assured that his preference for gardening over the evening news suits him just fine, while Alice may lie awake, ruminating over dire headlines, feeling the lonely burden of all that knowledge. Each might secretly envy the other's stance. Bob occasionally wonders if he should care more; Alice yearns for even a fraction of Bob's calm. Both are convinced the other is "doing life wrong." Yet each approach contains partial truths: Bob enjoys mental peace but lags in preparedness, while Alice's desire to stay informed could become self-defeating if it engulfs her in stress without leading to meaningful action.

Sometimes, selective ignorance shows up in daily misadventures. A friend declared they could ignore their car's gas light, confident they'd make it to the next station. They ended up stranded on a lonely stretch of road, phoning for help with an embarrassed laugh. Another colleague refused to open her electric bills for months in a bid to preserve her "financial Zen," only to discover a billing error that nearly led to a cutoff. Though these scenarios yield humorous stories, they also remind us that the hidden price of ignoring reality can be higher than the mental ease we temporarily gain.

That leads us to ask how we can protect ourselves from a perpetual downpour of bad news without letting ignorance become reckless. An "alien observer" trick, explored in the following chapter, can act as a middle ground, letting us see events from a wry or comedic distance rather than shutting them out altogether. When crises surge in the headlines, we can remain aware without letting them dominate our mental space to the point of constant dread. It is a reframing: acknowledging the problems yet refusing to be consumed by them. Instead of burying your head in the sand like an ostrich, you tilt your head slightly, watching with a calm vantage point that spares you the worst emotional fallout.

There is also the concept of an "information diet," analogous to a nutritional diet. As you balance proteins, carbs, and vitamins without overindulging in junk food, so too can you moderate your media consumption. Too much negative news fosters cynicism and helplessness; total ignorance can leave you dangerously disconnected. The ideal "diet" might blend credible sources in measured doses, set times of the day to read updates, and an exit strategy for when your anxiety alarm starts to ring. Think of it like "news vegetables" (essential facts) versus "news candy" (clickbait that triggers fear).

Humor can further soften the impact of distressing news. Some late-night TV shows or satire programs keep viewers informed while also injecting comedic detachment that can reduce despair. It isn't the same as not knowing, but it offers a gentler lens through which to process bleak headlines. If Alice could pepper her knowledge gathering with doses of wry commentary, she might relieve some of her tension, preserving enough mental space to act on what she learns, rather than just simmer in worry.

Eventually, the dinner party ends. Bob yawns, thanks the hosts, and heads home unperturbed. Alice lingers, preoccupied with the day's unsettling topics. Each sees the other as incomplete, yet both stances reflect coping styles that come with trade-offs. For most of us, a more balanced path feels healthiest. Yes, ignorance can bring short-term bliss during times of crisis overload. But knowledge, handled mindfully, can open the door to engagement, readiness, and even progress. The trick is to figure out where to draw the line.

Perhaps real peace emerges in accepting that life is messy and often beyond our control, so we grant ourselves mental breaks without forgoing all awareness. Socrates famously claimed he knew nothing, but he was not advocating blindness, rather a humble engagement with reality, aware that total mastery is unattainable. A person who recognizes they can't fix every crisis yet doesn't need to track each despairing event gains a genuine serenity that is neither naive nor paralyzing. There are times to dive in and times to stand back; that is the essence of wisdom.

Key Takeaways

- Ignorance can lower stress: In novel or overwhelming circumstances, being less informed sometimes results in higher happiness than being hyperaware (Kanazawa & Li, 2018).

- Long-term ignorance backfires: Problems don't vanish just because we ignore them; eventually, reality intrudes. We do better when we know enough to act on health or safety issues.

- Socratic humility: There's wisdom in recognizing what you don't know, rather than blindly avoiding knowledge.

Accepting uncertainty can bring peace without full-on denial.

- Selective ignorance: It's fine, helpful, even, to unplug from relentless information overload, as long as you remain open to crucial facts that help you take meaningful action.

In that sense, "ignorance is bliss" remains a paradox. In small doses, it can serve as a soothing escape from relentless negativity. Yet it also risks sliding into denial that undermines responsibility and sows bigger crises later. Finding a balanced sweet spot, staying adequately informed while preserving mental health, requires intention and self-awareness. In the next chapter, we shift beyond merely ignoring bad news to exploring how we can shift our perspective on routine stressors through humor and imaginative detachment. Where ignorance surrenders to not knowing, perspective chooses to see differently, potentially letting us stay open-eyed without losing our composure. For those who succeed in reframing, comedic distance might become the new "bliss", one that embraces reality but refuses to let it define our emotional state every waking hour.

The next Chapter 3 is the right place to discuss why perspective is everything. Instead of ignoring what frightens or stresses us, what if we could see it from a clever, comical, or outside viewpoint, thereby neutralizing much of its sting? To overcome our inherent biases in storytelling, we'll invite a guest, an "alien observer," whose perspective can transform daily annoyances into comedic material, allowing us to remain vigilant while maintaining sanity. Let's see.

Chapter 3: Perspective Is Everything

If you were an alien watching us, what on Earth would you think?

A friend once asked me once, "If you were an alien watching us, what on Earth would you think?" . That question has lingered with me. The vision of an inquisitive space creature, baffled by our practices, from the rite of drinking hot bean-water in the morning (coffee) to the grave observance of refreshing email every few moments, transforms mundane stress into the hilariously weird. This mental exercise might seem frivolous, but what it demonstrates is a deeper truth: adjusting our stance can transform how we feel.

Perspective doesn't equal avoidance, it means reapproaching it with a different lens. Whereas the phrase "ignorance is bliss" would have us skip or completely avoid certain truths, the art of perspective-taking is to recognize the facts and then shift the lens through which those facts view us, so they no longer loom larger than life. If you've ever walked away from an angry argument and thought how ridiculous it all sounded or read an old diary entry and chuckled at what felt at the time like the end of the world, then you've already tasted the strength of perspective. This chapter describes how intentionally switching our point of view, occasionally with humor, can reduce stress, ignite creativity and aid in navigating through life more gracefully.

Eyes from Space and Their Human Stage

The anthropological satire about the "Nacirema" tribe is frequently referenced in college textbooks as an example of how everyday behavior can become absurd when viewed from afar. "Nacirema" is simply "American" spelled backward, and the anthropologist Horace Miner portrayed normal U.S. behaviors, bathroom rituals, dental checkups, as if they were strange tribal practices. Students reading about "holy-mouth-men" (dentists) or "magical potions" (toothpaste) may not, at first, recognize these descriptions as torture for themselves. That moment of recognition is funny and illuminating: It shows how accustomed we are to some elements of our daily life that we take them for granted, just because we are so used to them.

Along the same lines, think about how children first respond to adult norms. To a toddler, it might be comical to watch adults congregate in offices, as they tap their fingers into laptops, or speak animatedly into rectangular devices pressed against their heads. It only loses its sense of novelty once we get used to it and stop questioning it. The "alien observer" perspective is basically a kind of childlike, anthropologist-style vantage point, noticing the hidden absurdity in everyday patterns. A lens from which humor comes, if we decide to take one.

I was reminded of an "alien test" that a good friend swears by whenever she's trapped in a spiral of what-ifs. If she's panicking about how she has exactly 427 unread emails, she imagines explaining email to an alien: "You see, we humans keep little rectangles of data in a glowing box, and, if the digital sum at the corner gets above 400, we lose sleep!" As soon as she starts to speak that reasoning aloud, she finds herself laughing. It provides comic distance, a way to free the mind from the chokehold. It wasn't like the number or amount of the email changed, but her relationship to it did.

The Power of Perspective: The Psychology of Distancing

Social psychologists and clinical researchers have extensively researched how reappraising your perspective can alleviate emotional distress. The theory of "psychological distance" (Trope & Liberman, 2011) has proposed that the farther the event is (be it in emotion, time, or space), the weaker our emotional response will be. For example, seeing a fictional drama about a tragedy usually hits less hard than reading a real-world account of that same tragedy. Or imagine reflecting on a minor heartbreak from your teenage years: The passage of time may render that once-devastating breakup almost endearing. By varying the distance, whether that be temporal or perceptual, we can often defuse a sense of crisis in the moment.

In therapeutic contexts, some techniques foster "self-distancing" or "observer perspectives" to help people cope with powerful emotions (Kross & Ayduk, 2011). Instead of replaying an upsetting moment from the first-person "I," a client could describe it as though she were reading the story of someone else, or in the third person: "She felt bad because..." Even a slight change in pronoun can lighten the emotional load, research on self-talk and coping has shown. When negative experiences arise, if we can rise outside of ourselves, if only for a moment, and for strategic purposes, we can respond more calmly.

We don't have to be in formal therapy to employ these insights. Humor is a built-in tool for distancing. When we laugh at a tense situation, such as a heated debate over which potato salad recipe is best at a family reunion, we are, in a sense, acknowledging the tension but refusing to let it overtake us. By framing the debate as a comically absurdist situation, "We're grown adults vigorously debating tuber and mayonnaise!", we allow a healthy, psychological distance that helps prevent stress overload."

Naturally, perspective is not a magic wand. Serious issues require real attention. But even in dark times, a light of "outside eyes" can sustain mental lucidity. Emergency responders and medical personnel often speak of cultivating a functional lack of attachment , viewing a crisis from a professional perspective in order to do their jobs efficiently. There's a time crunch, but maybe after the crisis, they'll process the emotional toll individually. That layered perspective keeps them calm in the chaos.

Everyday Application of the "Alien Observer" Trick

Looking at Commuting Woes Through a Different Lens

Traffic is a good overall stressor. Many of us have sat attired behind a row of cars, creeping forward in a scorching sun. If you picture an alien swinging through and saying, "Why do thousands of you clump together in metal boxes every morning, honking at each other as you trudge along at snail pace?" you might crack a smile. The reality of commuting is unchanged, but humor can help diffuse exasperation. You might think, "This is, really, so strange," and your rage might dissipate enough that you can address the logjam with a little more patience, maybe turn on some music or an audiobook you love as you wait.

Transforming Chores into Quirky Rituals

One friend refers to her weekend ritual of tidying up around the house "The Great House Safari." She pretends that the vacuum cleaner is her safari jeep, and she imagines every dusty corner as "uncharted territory." Silly? Absolutely. But that childlike reframing transforms the quotidian into a playful quest. Things once dreaded can grow more manageable. The "alien perspective" at work here is allowing you to look at common household chores in a new or funny way. You might not find it life changing, but if it brightens up the 45 minutes you spend cleaning, isn't that a minor victory?

Defusing Social Awkwardness

Social situations are fraught with embarrassment. From forgetting a name to fumbling on your words, moments like this can feel mortifying at the time. And then there's the idea of stepping outside of yourself, like a director watching the outtakes of a film. "Cut! Let's reshoot that introduction scene. No big deal." It can cause that awkwardness balloon to sag. The comedic reframe is a psychological shock absorber, telling you that a small snafu is part of the greater human farce, not a personal disaster.

When Perspective Fails, or Backfires

While changing your perspective can help, it's not a one-size-fits-all solution. Sometimes someone is trying to joke away a serious issue, trying to laugh off a real fight in a relationship or dismissing an urgent health concern as a running gag, thereby avoiding taking needed action. This is a danger of comedic distance: it can tip over into denial if it's used to avoid confrontation or change. We need to figure out whether the comic or "alien observer" approach is helping us clear our heads about the situation or just letting us skip the gloss-over phase.

Similarly, urging someone in crisis to step back to an outside perspective can sometimes come across as dismissive if done too early or without sufficient empathy. A bereaved person might not immediately be served by a kind of comedic reframing. It is all about timing and sensitivity. It is one thing to lighten one's own burdens by imagining the scenario from an alien point of view; it is another to impose that view on someone not yet prepared to accept it.

The temptation toward cynicism also looms. In some circles, it quickly becomes second nature to take a stance of perpetual detachment or irony, everything's a cosmic joke. That may diminish authentic engagement. If we view each problem as an amusing spectacle, we run the risk of failing ever to tackle systemic injustices or real tragedies that require empathy and action. At times, the attempt at perspective must move from comic detachment to deliberate engagement.

Perspective as a Fuel for Creativity

A hidden benefit of changing perspectives is that it fosters creativity. Many forms of breakthroughs, scientific, artistic and personal, come at moments when we recognize the territory we know well in new ways. There are many legendary anecdotes of an inventor or innovator, and they often center around someone breaking through mainstream thought. The psychologist Mihaly Csikszentmihalyi (1996) has commented on the frequent "reframing" of problems by creative minds, challenging assumptions that others take for granted.

Consider your own "Eureka!" moments. They frequently happen during mundane activities, when showering or mindlessly washing dishes. A major reason is that they're unguarded moments when your brain naturally shifts to an outsider vantage, re-linking ideas, connecting concepts from angles you would never consider. If we can take an alien observer perspective consciously, if only for brief periods of time, if we allow ourselves to observe a challenge as if for the first time, we can break thought patterns that have become rut-like and influence innovation.

This creative bonus is not limited to inventors or artists. Even mundane life decisions can be improved with a lighter touch: if a messy desk over time might benefit from a new organization structure, a staid volunteer committee process might be reworked to give life to a local charity event. By taking a step back, we avoid the trap of "this is how we've always done it.

The Funhouse Mirror Effect: Laughing at Ourselves

Like a funhouse mirror, comedic perspective exaggerates certain elements of our day-to-day behavior until they become absurd. We could cringe-laugh at how fervently we've scrolled through social media if it's packaged in the form of a sketch about neurotic characters glued to miniature screens. Psychologists say self-directed humor, making gentle, self-deprecating jokes, can be a way to embrace our flaws without shame (Martin, 2018). This is different from negative, belittling humor that cuts down oneself or other people. The healthful brand jokes about common foibles: "I spent 20 minutes looking for my glasses that were on my head the whole time, classic me!"

Then by identifying an overreaction or meltdown in comedic terms, saying, for example, that you had a panic attack that felt like "my brain hosting an impromptu clown festival at 2 A.M.", we sidle away from the emotional charge around the meltdown. We're not minimizing the anxiety; we're just naming it in a manner that gives a bit of a buffer. A funny description may suffice for recall, "Oh, this is a long-running production my mind likes to put on, but I can change the channel at some point."

We should not obviously treat debilitating mental health issues as just punch lines. A funhouse mirror approach is like salt and seasoning, applied sparingly to lighten our mental load. If more serious issues remain, professional assistance or more of a clinical therapeutic approach is advisable. But on a day-to-day basis, a sprinkle of humor, brought on by perspective, can help us avoid languishing in the weightiness of our own story.

Eyes of Alien and Our Theater of Human

The anthropological satire of the "Nacirema" tribe, often found in college textbooks to show how mundane behaviors can seem surreal from an outsider's viewpoint, traces back to Horace Miner's essay on U.S. cultural practices (Miner, 1956). "Nacirema" is simply "American" spelled backward, yet Miner wrote about everyday behaviors, such as bathroom habits or dental checkups, as though they were strange tribal rituals. Students reading about "holy-mouth-men" (dentists) or "magical potions" (toothpaste) may not initially realize that these descriptions apply to themselves. That moment of recognition is as funny as it is illuminating: it reveals how we often take certain parts of daily life for granted simply because we are so accustomed to them.

In much the same way, consider how children initially react to adult norms. A toddler may laugh upon watching adults congregate in offices, tapping away at keyboards, or speaking solemnly into small rectangular devices pressed to their ears. This fresh perspective soon fades as we grow used to it. The "alien observer" lens is essentially a childlike or anthropologist-like viewpoint, one that spots the inherent silliness in our habitual rhythms. Humor flows freely from there, if we choose to let it.

A good friend of mine relies on an "alien test" whenever she feels overwhelmed. If she's panicking about having precisely

427 unread emails, she imagines explaining email to a visiting extraterrestrial: "We humans store tiny rectangles of data in a glowing box, and once the corner number surpasses 400, we can't sleep!" The instant she tries to articulate that logic, she starts laughing. That satirical distance releases the mental grip. The total number of emails hasn't changed, but her relationship to them has.

Case Study: Zoorg's Weekend visit

Suppose, Zoorg, an alien guest spent the Weekend at your home. He invisibly studies you for the whole weekend hovering in the corner, taking precise notes about your habits. All of them, including the ones you only thought of:

Friday Night: You collapse on the couch, doomscrolling on your phone when you're not half-watching a show. Zoorg is unsure if the glowing device you hold in your palm has brain-melting magnetism. You pause, take a deep breath, and when Zoorg notes your occasional sigh or your furrowing brow, Zoorg makes a note of it: "Human spends hours on bright rectangle for quick emotional hits, very strange."

Saturday Morning: You throw yourself out of bed complaining that it's "too early," although it's already 9 A.M. Zoorg takes note of your sophisticated ritual: machinery makes (beeps) at you (alarm clock), you complain, and then you consume a vile brown bitter liquid (coffee) with total devotion.

Saturday Afternoon: You have been doing errands, and are now in traffic, cursing an endless line of cars backed up behind you. Zoorg sees identical metallic boxes creeping along, horns blaring haphazardly. "Why do they do this daily?" Zoorg wonders. "They seem to generate stress for themselves and then complain about the stress they've generated.

Saturday Night: Small talk with friends is repeated ad nauseam, smartphone checks are frequent, laughter shared over jokes that aren't really funny and complaints about bigger ills, politics, money, leading to mild arguments. Zoorg comments on the irony: humans want social bonding but tend to undermine it with arguments about abstract beliefs.

Sunday: You have a meltdown upon realizing the workweek starts soon. Zoorg addresses the phenomenon of "Sunday Scaries." You pace, fret that things aren't checked off lists, check email. Then you chill out by late afternoon to a comfort show. The last entry from Zoorg: "Human engages energy imagining future problems, bored and anxious simultaneously. "Possible comic contradiction?"

Zoorg's anthropological notes can bring a smile but also might make you think. None of your habits changed; through the perspective of an extraterrestrial researcher, however, you see the fundamental absurdity in rhythms you rarely acknowledge. This comic lens might spur you to change something, perhaps you institute a phone cut-off after dinner, or Sunday nights start to include a new ritual that helps to lessen the anxiety. Finding humor in your own habits allows you to be more open to improvement than would callous self-beratement.

Key Takeaways

- Perspective Changes Stress: When perception becomes comedic "alien observer," anxiety fades, and the absurdity behind why we do the things we do comes to light. This does not bypass real issues but rather reframes our emotional engagement with them.

- Psychological Distance Reduces Emotional Intensity: Research indicates that creating psychological distance can reduce emotional intensity. For example, adopting a third-person perspective, imagining a memory from outside one's body, or even using light humor to "rename" an anxiety "character" may diminish the force of distressing emotions (Kross & Ayduk, 2011; Trope & Liberman, 2011)

- Funny as Self-Distancing: Jibes at your own weaknesses can dilute negative feelings and palliative the pains, if you continue to notice and care about serious needs.

- Creativity Boosts: New Vistas: Changing your perspective helps you get out of mental ruts, leading to insight and problem-solving in both personal and professional situations (Csikszentmihalyi, 1996)

- Don't be Too Distant: Too much comedic distance can easily go toward denialism or cynicism. Balance is essential, perspective should clarify, not obfuscate, serious issues that need addressing.

- Conflict Navigation: Short periods of outside perspective can ease heated arguments, lower defensiveness and encourage empathy by exposing the sometimes-comical nature of our disagreements.

Perspective is not just for self-reflection; it's essential for resolving conflicts, as well. Imagine a spat between family members over holiday plans. Both sides feel they are being personally attacked. If one person takes a step back for a minute, maybe viewing the ruckus with an imaginary television studio audience camera, they can appreciate the comic irony: "We're yelling about who's bringing mashed potatoes and who gets there at 2:00 vs. 2:15." Realizing that outside perspective might motivate them to crack a light joke ("Hey, if the potatoes are five minutes late, the world's not going to end!"). That flash of humor, rooted in perspective, would be enough to diffuse tension and pivot back towards productive solutions.

Of course, not all conflicts are petty. Some are based on longstanding issues. But even then, changing perspective can help people on each side of the divide realize that the other side's perspective makes sense, from their "internal camera." If I were them, how would I see me right now? fosters empathy. Comedic reframing won't solve massive divides overnight, but it can reduce the emotional heat in a situation and allow reason and empathy to re-enter the conversation.

"Perspective is everything" may be a well-worn cliché, but it persists because reframing how we look at a problem typically does more than an outward adjustment ever could. Ignoring trouble might have left us unprepared (as we saw in Chapter 2), but reframing trouble might leave us informed and lighter and less burdened by panic. Like donning a pair of slapstick spectacles, comedic distance remakes anxiety into a riddle we can greet rather than a tempest that roils us nonstop.

We don't need to be jesters in our own lives full-time; at times, seriousness is deserved. But if we can assume, even for a moment, the perspective of an alien observer or a wise outsider, we might find a reserve of resolve. In the next chapter, we'll change the subject from vantage points to the connection between money and happiness, another area of life where illusion, presumption and a shift in perspective are in abundance. Can perspective help us grapple with that ageless debate about whether money can buy happiness, or is that a puzzle unto itself? Let's find out. While perspective is everything, the next Chapter 4, spices things up discussing the diversion perspectives of Money Can't Buy Happiness. Or can it?

Chapter 4: Money Can't Buy Happiness. Or

Can It?

"No, money doesn't make you happy. But it can get you a yacht big enough to sail right up next to it," quipped singer David Lee Roth (cited in several interviews, though never in a clearly cited single written source). This cheeky observation crystallizes a long-debated axis in philosophy, culture and social science: Does wealth bring well-being, or is it an illusion that puts us on a hamster wheel of upwelling dissatisfaction? And like many a rejoinder on the subject, it mellows the beloved receive into "money can't buy happiness" with a wily admission that money can at least make life more cushioned yet serves as no panacea.

Despite throwing around proverbs such as "Money can't buy love" and "The best things in life are free" in our everyday life, we also say things like "I'd rather cry in a Ferrari than on a bicycle" when we hit moments of cynicism. Underneath the humor is a very real question: Where does money's influence on happiness begin, and where does it end? This chapter addresses that question from several angles: the so-called happiness-income plateau; real life cases of lottery winners and losers; philosophic musings; and scientific findings about spending habits. The result is a nuanced exploration that reveals money isn't a golden ticket to happiness, but neither is it beside the point. As with many things in life, the answer is a little complex.

Revisiting the $75,000 "Happiness Plateau"

A critical inflection point in the mainstream conversation came with a study from Princeton led by Daniel Kahneman (Nobel laureate, economics) and Angus Deaton that reported that Americans' day-to-day emotional well-being appeared to plateau somewhere above $75,000 per year (Kahneman & Deaton, 2010). This number circulated quickly, in part because it was so specific and could be easily recalled. The blogosphere exploded with pieces declaring "Once you earn $75k, more money won't help you!, which some interpreted as a near-universal law of happiness. It surely appealed to those who prefer a neat, tidy answer to the perennial question, "When is enough enough?"

However, that original conclusion was based on specific measures of "emotional well-being" and on data that had some limitations, like being mainly about the United States and being self-reports. Gradually, as more data came in from diverse populations and methodologies were honed, scholars started to suspect that the mythical $75k cap was overly simplistic. In 2023, an updated paper by Kahneman, alongside researcher Matthew Killingsworth, reexamined the question using more extensive and more granular datasets (Killingsworth, Kahneman, & Mellers, 2023). Their findings suggested that happiness keeps increasing above $75k, well into six-figure salaries for most people.

Yet there was a nuance: People who are very unhappy for other things (like illness, marital strife or other life crises) don't necessarily experience persistent increases of happiness from higher sums of income. In that sub-sample, well-being increased with income only up to a point of ~$100k and then plateaued. Yet for most, there was still (diminishing) gain as income increased, even up to $500k in the sample. "If you're rich and miserable, more money won't help; for everyone else, it does," (Killingsworth et al., 2023).

What does this mean in practical terms? First, it implies that money still has a moderate ability to buy happiness, at least if you're not in the grips of crippling personal or psychological problems. But the second reason is that the increases are smaller in magnitude as you move up the income scale, and once you cross certain thresholds, other things, health, relationships, meaningful work, become much more important. The distinction between earning $50k and $100k is usually much bigger, in terms of decreasing stress/worry, than between the $550k and $600k, which is more of a slight upgrade in discretionary spending (or a little more inflating in savings).

What about the earlier claims that money becomes "Monopoly money" to your brain above a middle-class threshold? The new view is more nuanced: each extra dollar does tend to buy more happiness, but the marginal impact is smaller. That is, the "bang for your buck" diminishes. What feels like a lifesaver earning an extra $1,000 at $40k is often a shrug at $400k. And more to the point, how you get, and use, those better resources can make a huge difference to well-being, as we'll explore at length.

Perspectives of Wealth

Long before psychologists began churning out regression models and p-values, philosophers, religious teachers and folk wisdom addressed the question of money's place in a good life. "Money is a good servant but a bad master," says an old saying, reflecting the struggle between using money figuratively as a tool and allowing it to dictate your life. Ancient Greek thinkers were often concerned with moderation: Aristotle, for example, argued that prosperity (including material wealth) helps humans achieve something he called "eudaimonia" (which translates as human flourishing), but only when paired with virtue and wisdom.

Across cultures, meanwhile, you'll encounter admonitions about the hollowness of greed, from Lao Tzu's "He who knows he has enough is rich" (n.d.) to the Christian proverb that the love of money is the "root of all evil." The tension comes because money can, indeed, open doors, pay for an education, create art, feed the hungry, but if you allow it to pervade your mind, you risk losing sight of other aspects of life. And other very wealthy people indeed say they feel vacuous or wonder whether their wealth has shielded them from authentic human intimacy.

Data-driven research has all sorts of modern tendencies, but in general they echo these ancient findings: money generally does good where it alleviates suffering from poverty and allows autonomy, but beyond a certain point, you need to use it wisely, or you'll be as miserable as the next person, just in a gilded cage.

Lottery Winners and Losers

No scenario may better encapsulate the money-happiness paradox than that of lottery winners. If treasure were the path to everlasting happiness, these people would presumably be the happiest of the bunch. But media accounts typically dwell on "lottery curse" horror stories: winners who go bankrupt, socially ostracized or even killed. Though anecdotal, these narratives remind that millions in windfall can be psychologically destabilizing, if you're not prepared for it. One of the studies, from 1978 is often mentioned in this context, and it wasn't only lottery winners (Brickman et. al., 1978). It did find that lottery winners, after a period of initial euphoria, did not sustain significantly greater day-to-day happiness compared with a control group and even took less pleasure in mundane activities. At the same time, people who had become paraplegics due to accidents expressed less overall happiness than anyone else, but still not as low as you might expect, in part because of the human capacity for adaptation and the search for meaning. From this perspective, the emotional "high" of victory (or the emotional "low" of catastrophe) tends to back to baseline over time, a phenomenon known as the "hedonic treadmill" or "set-point" theory.

But newer work complicates this story. Some large jackpot winners use their winnings with prudence, investing mindfully, reflecting on personal relationships or using their winnings to pursue philanthropic causes, and report higher life satisfaction, in some cases for decades. A massive Swedish study reported long-term, improved mental well-being for people who had won big in the lottery, against some dire stories (Cesarini et al., 2016). So, which is correct? Both: If money serves your deeper wants, if it creates the experiences, you value, if it enables you to forge and maintain social bonds, it can enhance happiness; if it just amplifies bad decisions or brings predatory relatives out of the woodwork, it can plunge you into misery.

There are two potential winners one could consider being: Jane and John. Jane goes all-in on conspicuous consumption, mansions, sports cars, lavish parties, and attempts to buy loyalty from dozens of acquaintances. She's eventually consumed by her obligations to the upkeep of the multifamily properties, mismanages the finances, is paranoid of everyone who may want to get a piece of her fortune. Over time, she longs for her simpler life, when she was sure who her friends were. John, on the other hand, invests wisely, downshifts his work years (but not his work), allocates some winnings toward meaningful vacations or charitable projects, and feels more stable. Five years later, Jane is less happy than she was, while John reports a sustained increase in satisfaction.

Money is like a magnifying glass in that way: it magnifies what is already inside you, whether it's generosity and purpose and good planning or insecurity, impulsiveness and shallow relationships. In fact, money can buy a certain type of happiness or satisfaction, if it's used to purchase experiences, free time or investments in health and relationships. If employed simply for status or indulging every passing fancy, it may offer temporary pleasure but will likely fall short of creating lasting well-being.

Poverty, Riches, and Everything in Between

It would be reckless to assert that money doesn't matter in the slightest. Chronic stress in this way is a strong predictor of unhappiness, and the lack of money to meet one's own, often basic, needs (food, shelter, health care) creates chronic stress. Beginning in the 1970s, economist Richard Easterlin demonstrated that, on average, wealthier individuals report more happiness than poorer individuals in any given country (Easterlin, 1974). But when measuring change over time, the "Easterlin Paradox" more emerge. Older countries became wealthier, but average happiness didn't necessarily rise in a straight line, implying adaptation or rising expectations.

Still, reducing poverty makes a huge difference in well-being: If you can't pay rent or ensure your children have enough to eat, a pay raise or government assistance can dramatically improve day-to-day life. Too, vast wealth introduces a different set of afflictions. Trust problems, social isolation, or a lack of purpose can plague super-rich celebrities or tech entrepreneurs when their most immediate needs become more than satisfied. Of course, The Notorious B.I.G.'s money wisdom classic "Mo Money, Mo Problems" (1997) may be overstating things, but it conveys a correct impression that money can bring anxieties, fear of losing it, suspicion of others' motives, pressure to invest wisely.

The human mind naturally focuses on the 20% beyond what it already has in income as the source of "real" happiness. The 20% solution feels great in the moment, but we adapt, and again we desire that next uptick. This cyclical pursuit is called the "hedonic treadmill," a term that, along with the notion of a "set-point" for happiness, turns out to be limited in its use. So now instead of worrying about $$, you get used to new comforts and what was once wild becomes routine. Without some strategies, such as practicing gratitude or consciously telling ourselves to remember how far we've come, our brains can continue putting one more thing beyond our grasp.

One humorous note: those extreme penny pinchers who love clipping coupons may seem to derive as much pleasure from saving money as others do from spending it more lavishly. Not spending, then, becomes a small "treat" in itself, triggering a hit of dopamine. Others don't experience that buzz until later, after a binge of consumption, such as a five-star meal, or a new gadget. Both show that money does not have a linear path to happiness, or a single pathway to happiness, universally. Knowing what matters most to you, experiences, security, philanthropy, or whatever, is what transforms everything.

Why Spending Wisely Matters

How much a household spends enters income as well and arguably matters as much (or more than) pure income. Prosocial spending or using money to benefit others through charity or gift-giving, is a greater driver of subjective well-being than spending money on oneself (Dunn, Aknin, & Norton, 2008). In fact, purchases of experiences (such as a once-in-a-lifetime trip or an immersion in a hobby) tend to deliver more lasting happiness than those involving material goods, which are soon relegated to the background. Psychologists instead consider experiences as more "socially connecting" and less susceptible to hedonic adaptation.

Equally, paying to "borrow time" can be a powerful happiness hack. It's yet another reason to hire someone to do your unwanted chores, housecleaning, lawn-mowing, saving you hours for more meaningful or enjoyable things. If you're juggling three jobs to stay afloat, more money could very well lower stress by allowing you to quit one job, thus optimizing sleep and mental health. But if you're already financially secure and decide to spend your money on a more expensive car rather than liberating time or supporting your personal values, you may discover the new vehicle only contributes marginally to your pleasure.

In other words, it's not money, per se, that leads to contentment; it's spending money in ways that reflect your values, your passions and your social ties. If you derive personal joy from traveling with loved ones or starting a community project, spending time and resources in that area may indeed lead to greater well-being than mindlessly accumulating possessions.

The Adaptation Conundrum

Even if you're very careful with your spending, you still can't escape adaptation. From the good to the bad, humans, bless our hearts, can get used to just about anything. That phenomenon, known as "hedonic adaptation," is exactly what the 1978 lottery winner study was designed to draw attention to (Brickman et al., 1978). The house of your dreams, a year into living in it, may not grant you that daily jolt that you once hoped it would; your new $500-enabled smartphone quickly transforms into last year's model in your mind by this fall.

It is a double-edged adaptation. It, in a way, protects us from overwhelming despair after tragic happenings (paraplegia, to take one example). On the other hand, it prevents us from sustained euphoria after windfalls or large purchases, impelling us to pursue the next "upgrade." The only way to mitigate this treadmill is with purposeful practice, gratitude exercises, volunteering, at least rotating your luxuries so that any given one doesn't become a mundane fact of life. So, if you get a fancy sports car, only drive it on the weekend or during special occasions so it's an event rather than your daily commute vehicle.

Philosophical lines of thought around the world, from Stoicism in ancient Greece to Buddhism in Asia, have taught some iteration of the idea that craving leads to dissatisfaction. Money fueling loads of desires can escalate that dissatisfaction very fast. If we are not careful. This doesn't mean that living in ascetic poverty is the way to joy; it does mean we must treat resources with care, aware that adaptation and rising expectations is hardwired into our brains.

Emotional Security versus Chasing Status

In happiness economics, a major difference is between relieving negative feelings (say, stress about bills) and eliciting positive emotions (such as excitement, pride, or status to be had from major purchases). Liberty from pocket-to-pocket dwelling pays a mental health dividend. But once you have some stability, motivation to continue scaling the income ladder may come from comparing yourself to peers, or the desire for status symbols. Studies show that happiness is very sensitive to social comparison: If you're earning $100k but all your close friends and family members earn $200k, you're likely going to feel inferior, whereas if you're earning $70k but your social circle is making $50k, you may feel relatively rich.

The trouble with status-based contentment is that it's precarious, it relies on outside reference points that can change as soon as you meet new people or move to a wealthier neighborhood. This is why some high-income earners keep clamoring for more. It disgusts comes not because you know that $200k or $500k isn't enough in an absolute scale, but someone else has more or they've simply mentally moved the bar. Here's where intangible factors, deep relationships, meaningful work, enriching growth, play a role, often outweighing the importance of raw net worth when you're above a base level of comfort.

Humor and Cultural Commentary

There's an unmistakable comic strip quality to how humans handle money. Think of the old line, "I'm not materialistic, I just like to have enough money to buy what I want." It is a winky admission that, although we talk about our higher purposes, a lot of us have a material itch we are happy to scratch, be it the shoes or the gadgets or the fancy coffee makers. One comedic example could be the "bargain-hunter's high", the inebriated rush of victory at discovering a dress that's 50 percent off. We may say ironically, "I saved $100 today when I purchased these discounted items," playing down that we still spent $200 to begin with.

In similar vein, there are endless comedic references to "frugal millionaires", the billionaires who continue to wear ratty jeans or who drive a 10-year-old car. Some for modesty and others because they truly despise waste. The contradiction between the net worth and the way the person spends, or lives life often invites questions or chuckles. Is that thriftiness a moral position, or simply old habits that never wore off? The jokes almost write themselves: "If I had a billion dollars, I would still order the $4.99 burger combo. It's called principle... and a discount coupon.

After all, these whimsical insights remind us that money is rooted in our quirks and our culture. One person's "over-the-top" indulgence is another person's everyday living. Someone else's "cheapskate approach" might the savvy path to less money stress. This comedic dimension helps us understand that rules about money and happiness are rarely "one-size-fits-all."

Perhaps a Balanced Perspective

Money isn't everything. But it's also not nothing. That tension encapsulates centuries of thinking on the subject, and the mountains of modern research corroborate it. To the extent that people are no longer straining to get by or can afford the basics, their quality of life can vastly improve, especially for those who in the past struggled with poverty. And for many of us, income boosts of $5k or so can continue to climb the scale of satisfaction above the much exalted $75k threshold.

But it's a game of diminishing returns. As income increases, you get less happiness for each dollar spent. And if you're unhappily ill, in an awful relationship or in dire psychological straits, more money won't necessarily solve that, at least, not directly. How you deploy your wealth is just as important. Purchases to foster experiences, relationships, philanthropy or to purchase your time back provide more consistent enhancement of well-being than burning cash on continuous status enhancements.

The amusing quips about crying in a Ferrari vs. a bicycle reveal our ambivalence: a nice seat and air conditioner might mitigate some of the crying, but not the actual reason we're crying. As we make our way through life, it can help to keep in mind that money is a tool, a powerful, necessary tool at times, but one that can eclipse much more important things in life if we become too consumed by it.

So maybe the path of least regret is that of earning enough to have enough, which lines up with our basic values, and then learning gratitude and intentionality about the excess. And if, after all that, we still want the Ferrari? At least we know we're purchasing it, eyes open, knowing that the real joy may be found less in the power under the hood and more in the ride, say, a weekend road trip with friends.

Key Takeaways

- Money and happiness are correlated: Generally, wealthier people are happier up to very high-income levels; there is no strict $75k happiness cap for most folks. However, gains in happiness per dollar diminish as income rises.

- Poverty hurts happiness: Lack of money for basic needs causes stress and unhappiness. Alleviating financial insecurity yields significant well-being improvements – money does buy the absence of misery in this case.
- Lottery outcomes vary: Some winners end up unhappy due to poor management or social fallout, while many maintain or increase life satisfaction. Money is a magnifier – it can magnify problems or opportunities.
- Spending wisely matters: Using money for experiences, personal growth, and helping others tends to produce more happiness than splurging on status goods. Money can "buy happiness" if it's spent in line with one's values (e.g. buying time or security).
- Adaptation is powerful: People adapt to wealth. After basic comfort is achieved, more money brings smaller boosts and one's expectations rise. Gratitude and purpose become crucial for happiness, whether one is middle-class or a millionaire.

Money isn't a guaranteed ticket to happiness, but it isn't irrelevant either. It's a bit like fuel for a car: you need enough to drive towards your happiness goals, but beyond a full tank, extra fuel won't make the journey more enjoyable (and carrying too much might even slow you down!). With this nuanced view, we can avoid idolizing money as a cure-all or dismissing it as meaningless. As we proceed, keep in mind how this theme might connect with other life truths. The next Chapter 5, we are getting deer to see how we understand the chaos in our heads, and what happens after that.

Chapter 5: Understanding the Chaos

The mind is like a circus: dazzling, frantic, and a little wild. Befriend the clowns, and the show becomes way less scary.

It was some time after 11 P.M. on a Tuesday, an arbitrary day in an ongoing week, that I became aware, how little I understood why, night after night, my brain was compelled to keep recycling a half-dozen worries on an infinite loop. I was sitting on my couch clutching a pillow shaped like a burrito (don't ask, long story), hearing fears scrawled in a panic repeat over and over: "What if my boss thinks I'm terrible?" "What if I didn't lock the door?" "What if that strange pain in my shoulder is a rare muscle disease?" If that sounds tiring, believe me, it was. It was as if the inside of my head was a three-ring circus, full of ringmaster (my overactive brain), trapeze artists (wild jumps of thought), and clowns (who showed up with scary or self-deprecating surprises). I'd used (or, I should say, refused to use) it for years, hoping it would go away, but after the grocery store panic attack I'll always remember, I decided enough was enough. If I wanted any peace, I needed to pull open the circus tent flap and see what was happening inside.

The First Peek Behind the Curtain

A few days after that meltdown in the store aisle, I'd fled, leaving a half-filled cart, I was sitting on the edge of my seat, nervous, in the waiting room of a therapist's office. I was messing with the zipper on my jacket, not looking at old magazines about gardening or celebrities. I had never been to a therapist, and half expected a stern Freudian with a monotone voice to tell me to lie down and rattle on about repressed childhood memories. To my surprise, Dr. Nguyen greeted me in a Star Wars T-shirt, handed me a cup of tea and smiled gently, as though saying, "We're in this together." More a supportive friend than a gatekeeper of mental secrets, she looked as if she could have made time within her schedule to read this piece of his life. I instantly relaxed, perhaps five percent, but in the universe of anxiety, that five percent is gold.

In that first session, after I rambled about how everything felt like it was imploding in my life, Dr. Nguyen said something that resonated: "Anxiety throws a lot of smoke bombs. A piece of therapy is to learn to see through the smoke and determine what is true." The idea that not everything my mind churns out is automatically true was revolutionary for me. I'd gotten accustomed to believing every panicky or negative thought, as if getting special bulletins from a willful (if paranoid) oracle. Dr. Nguyen's comment left open the possibility that the frantic messages in my mind might be illusions or half-truths.

Over the next few weeks, I learned that anxiety wasn't alone in my mental circus. I had more therapy sessions and during the exercises I started identifying the main "acts" that were roaming around in my head. The greatest act was anxiety, like a trapeze artist swinging at a height that seemed fatal with one misstep. Apparently, I had been living with generalized anxiety for years without naming it. I'd panic that I had left the stove on (even though I hadn't been cooking that day), or that my colleagues harbored an intense hatred for me, or that the small mole on my arm was skin cancer, my brain was professional when it came to fabricating catastrophes. Each fear careened into the next in a dizzying whir, never stopping long enough for me to catch my breath. It's no wonder I was zapped emotionally. "Another part of the show was Catastrophic Thinking, like a special effects department that turned any slightly concerning event into a full-blown "life is over" scenario. The phrase "We need to talk" from a boss or friend translated in my head to "I'm about to be fired, and soon I'll be homeless, living under a bridge with raccoons for neighbors." Then there was the Inner Critic Clown, who specialized in tossing pies of self-doubt: "Wow, look at you crying in a grocery store aisle. You're pathetic!" If you're thinking, "That's a bit harsh," trust me, it was.

Realizing that my mind's cast of characters wasn't me, just mental habits, was oddly empowering. One evening, wrapped in my burrito-blanket again, I doodled a little circus tent in my journal and began listing the big performers: The Worrier, The Critic, The Perfectionist, The Overthinker, The People-Pleaser, etc. I gave them all silly names, scribbled clown noses, and tried to imagine them as comedic archetypes rather than fearsome inner tyrants. It felt childish but, at the same time, delightfully freeing. I was turning intangible anxieties into cartoonish figures. The next time a wave of dread hit me, like "Oh no, my friend didn't text me back; she must hate me!", I visualized that as the Overthinker swinging onto the stage. Labeling the intrusion forced me to say, "Wait, is that rational?" and sometimes, I'd even muster a half-smile.

Mapping the Mind's Terrain

Understanding the circus acts took me deeper into the realm of psychology. Dr. Nguyen introduced me to the idea that thoughts are just thoughts, not objective truths set in stone (Beck, 1976). Cognitive-behavioral therapy (CBT) emphasizes that we can learn to notice our thoughts, evaluate them, and replace or modify the unhelpful ones. For me, this concept was like switching on the lights in a haunted house. The jump-scare ghosts might still be there, but now I could see they were just cardboard cutouts and special effects rather than real poltergeists.

I began reading articles on anxiety and depression and how adrenaline floods your body when you perceive a threat, even if it's just an email alert. Realizing that my pounding heart and sweating during panic were, in fact, normal bodily reactions to perceived danger (no matter how trivial that "danger" was) helped reduce some of the terror. Physiology wasn't the enemy; it was simply overreacting to false alarms.

Simultaneously, I encountered the concept of cognitive distortions, tricky, distorted ways our brains interpret events (Burns, 1989; Beck & Emery, 1985). My personal highlight reel included catastrophizing, all-or-nothing thinking, "Either I do this perfectly or I'm a hopeless failure", mind reading. "She thinks I'm annoying, I just know it", fortune telling "This meeting will definitely be humiliating", and personalization, "Those people laughing near me must be mocking me". Gaining familiarity with these distortions gave me a sort of "cheat sheet" for my mental patterns. Instead of feeling helpless when gloom descended, I could label it: "Oh, hey, that's catastrophizing again." This labeling alone didn't erase the anxiety, but it created a precious pause, a window where I could challenge the distortion or at least refuse to let it run the whole show.

Therapy for me included some CBT exercises, such as writing down a dreaded scenario. "My boss said she needs to see me this afternoon!" and exploring alternative explanations or more balanced thoughts ("She may want to clarify a task or provide normal feedback. She didn't sound angry. She also praised me last week for finishing a project."). Forcing myself to do this on paper felt clumsy at first, like I was fighting a long-standing reflex. But with repetition, it became easier to spot the leaps in logic. The mental muscle I was building was the ability to question my thoughts rather than instantly bow to them.

Small Victories in the Daily Chaos

I remember one afternoon at work. My boss told me she had some notes on a report. Naturally, my mind jumped to "She hated it. I failed. I bet she regrets hiring me." This time, though, I recognized the cast: the Inner Critic and Catastrophic Thinking bounding onto the stage. I paused and forced myself to rewrite the scenario: "She had suggestions for improvement, which is normal. It doesn't mean I've failed. In fact, she said 'good work' overall before diving into changes, maybe I should focus on that." Catching the distortion felt like a small victory, but an empowering one. I was still anxious, but at least I wasn't spiraling into meltdown territory.

This process didn't solve everything overnight. Even after weeks of therapy, I'd still catch my mind veering into doomsday territory. But being able to map out the "circus acts" gave me a sense of orientation. Anxiety or catastrophic thoughts might appear, but I could label them, anticipate their favorite times to pop up (like 2 A.M. when I was too wired to sleep), and prepare coping strategies, like deep breathing (Brown & Gerbarg, 2009) or journaling. Over time, I realized the anxious mind thrives on confusion and stealth; naming it and shining a light on it was like thwarting an ambush. Hard to get fully blindsided by Wendy the Worrier if you see her sprinting toward you waving a big sign that says, "Impending Doom, Act Now!"

The Role of Journaling and Self-Reflection

One of the most transformative daily habits I adopted was journaling. Initially, I wrote only when anxious thoughts swarmed, but soon I found that a brief 10-minute writing session each night drastically reduced my mental clutter. Research indicates that expressive writing or journaling can decrease anxiety, improve mood, and even support physical health (Baikie & Wilhelm, 2005; Medical News Today, 2023). I'd often start an entry with, "Time: 11 p.m., Mood: anxious, Thoughts: replaying conversation with coworker, certain I sounded dumb." Then, examining the evidence, I'd see how fleeting or illogical that worry might be. Or I'd at least catch a pattern, like noticing my anxieties spike late at night when I'm tired. Over time, these notes revealed recurring themes, which eventually made them less convincing. You can't trick yourself with the same illusion a hundred times once you've documented it.

Journaling also gave me a safe space to rant or be ridiculous on paper, like describing Catastrophic Thinking as a cheesy movie trailer voice: "In a world where one email could mean total destruction, only one person can cringe themselves to death…" Silly, yes, but laughter can be a powerful disruptor of anxiety. I'd often read my own comedic meltdown scripts the next day and think, "Wow, that's entertaining in a weird way, but not exactly plausible."

Adventures in Mindfulness

Another technique Dr. Nguyen recommended was mindfulness, something I'd heard a lot about but always suspected was too "zen" for my frantic mind. Mindfulness, in essence, is paying attention to the present moment without judgment (Kabat-Zinn, 1990). That might sound too gentle to handle the juggernaut of anxiety, but it turned out to be surprisingly helpful. One simple exercise was to imagine my thoughts as leaves drifting down a stream. As each anxious thought arose, "I'll fail tomorrow's presentation", I'd label it, place it on a leaf, and watch it float by. I didn't fight or analyze it; I simply let it pass. This separated me from the immediate panic, giving me a vantage point on the bank. At first, I got swept into the water every 12 seconds, but with practice, I learned to remain more of an observer (Kabat-Zinn, 1990; Segal, Williams, & Teasdale, 2013).

Was it a miracle cure? No. But each mindful moment felt like a brief reprieve from the mental chatter. Over time, those moments added up. Instead of feeling like a hapless spectator at my own mental circus, I became something akin to the circus manager who recognized each act and decided how long it would perform. Not total control, but much improved compared to letting the clowns run wild.

The Power of Talking It Out

Therapy remained the linchpin of my progress. Yet, I also discovered that talking to trusted friends or family members, people who had the empathy or humor to say, "I've been there too!", helped normalize what I was experiencing. Sometimes, we'd share replays of our anxious brains: "I was sure my boss was glaring at me because of that late email. Turns out she was just squinting at her phone." Hearing these parallels eased the sense of isolation. Humans are wired for connection, and anxiety often thrives in isolation, telling you that you're uniquely defective. Finding out that others also had meltdown thoughts about a random comment gave me comfort.

Still, an important caveat is that not everyone is equipped to handle your confessions. Some might unintentionally dismiss your worries: "Don't be silly, you're overreacting." Others might feed the panic: "Oh wow, that's definitely serious." It helps to identify the safe listeners, those who respond with understanding or a gentle comedic reframe. Dr. Nguyen sometimes called it "co-regulation," the notion that we can borrow calm from supportive relationships, much like an infant is soothed by a caregiver's steady presence (Schore, 2019).

Humor as a Deflector Shield

One of my favorite personal coping tricks was comedic self-talk. I'd imagine my anxiety as a cartoon character or a flamboyant announcer. Example: If I felt on edge about not replying to an email quickly, I'd imagine a ring announcer voice: "Ladies and gentlemen, in this corner, we have Felicity's Anxiety, wearing the bright pink robe of imaginary deadlines, claiming she must respond this second or face humiliation!" That slight shift in tone, making it silly, took the panic from a 9 down to maybe a 6. Because it's hard to be petrified when you're chuckling.

Numerous studies suggest humor can help alleviate stress, improve mood, and even strengthen the immune system (Martin, 2018; Gelkopf, 2011). Of course, humor has to be used wisely, it's not a license to trivialize genuine pain. But in my personal journey, gentle mockery of my overblown fears served as a release valve. Instead of letting anxiety posture as unstoppable doom, I'd grin and say, "Sure, Catastrophizer, keep talking. You're entertaining, but I see you're still wearing those clown pants."

Embracing Anxiety Without Letting It Drive

A significant lesson emerged: Trying to eradicate all anxiety was futile, maybe even counterproductive. Anxiety, at its core, can be a protective mechanism, alerting us to potential dangers. But in my case, it was stuck in overdrive, freaking out about everything from job performance to weird insect bites. Once I stopped demonizing anxiety altogether, I found a healthier stance: acceptance with boundaries. I could say to my anxious mind, "Look, I hear you. You're worried about potential humiliation at the meeting. That's normal. But you don't get to run the entire day."

This approach is reminiscent of Acceptance and Commitment Therapy (ACT), which teaches that refusing to feel anxiety often backfires, making anxiety stronger (Hayes, Strosahl, & Wilson, 2012). Instead, you acknowledge anxious feelings, like circus clowns, and gently direct them to the side stage so you can carry on. Over time, the clowns might quiet down or at least disrupt your show less.

Observations in Retrospect

Now, as I reflect on that old sense of chaos in my mind, I see it with less dread and more curiosity. I can appreciate the flamboyance of the mental acts: Anxiety as the trapeze artist, the Catastrophizer as the special effects wizard, the Inner Critic as a snarky clown. None of them truly define me. They're just mental patterns, shaped by past experiences, biology, and personal habits. With therapy, self-awareness, journaling, mindfulness, supportive conversations, and yes, humor, I've learned to manage them. I can't evict them from the circus entirely, but I can prevent them from swinging wildly without safety nets.

Over months, I realized something: The mind's chaos isn't necessarily a sign I'm "broken." It can also be a source of creativity, empathy, and depth. We often conflate anxiety with weakness, but when harnessed, that sensitivity might help me notice subtle details or approach projects with thoroughness. The trick is to keep it regulated, to let the anxious mind serve as a watchful sentinel rather than a shrieking alarm 24/7.

Understanding the chaos in our heads is half the battle. Once you identify the "circus acts" in your mind, they become less mysterious and more workable. Dr. Nguyen's metaphor of "seeing through the smoke bombs" remains a vivid reminder that anxious illusions, while convincing, are often just illusions. My mental circus has not folded its tent, but it's a more organized show these days, with me in the director's seat rather than a terrified spectator.

If your own mind sometimes feels like a carnival gone rogue, consider shining a light on each performer. Maybe you'll spot a tangle of worry-based illusions that can be gently teased apart with humor and self-awareness. Maybe you'll discover a hidden well of resilience once you see how your anxious thoughts are just "characters," not your core identity. And who knows, you might even find a comedic edge in describing your mental show. After all, laughter doesn't solve every problem, but it sure can stop a menacing clown from seeming too scary.

Reading back on my journey, I recall nights of frantic journaling, therapy sessions filled with "Aha!" moments, and comedic inner monologues that made me giggle in the midst of panic. I hope that sharing these experiences shows that while the path isn't always linear, ups, downs, and sideways loops are normal, the chaos can be understood, if never fully tamed, in ways that restore your sense of agency and humor.

Key Takeaways

- Your thoughts are not always truth: Our minds can play tricks (cognitive distortions). Recognizing these patterns is the first step to defusing them.
- Name your mental "characters": Externalizing anxiety or negative thoughts (e.g., giving your inner critic a funny name) helps you see them as separate from your core self.
- Journaling reveals patterns: Writing anxious thoughts helps you spot recurring worries. Seeing them on paper can make you realize, "Oh, it's this thing again."
- Learn the science/psychology: Understanding the chemical and cognitive roots of anxiety turns a mysterious enemy into a known challenge.
- Mindfulness of thoughts creates distance: Practices that treat thoughts as passing phenomena can reduce overthinking and panic over time.

- Humor can disarm fear: Gently mocking your anxious thoughts (with kindness) can lessen their impact and remind you they're not invincible.

But by the time I finished my self-discovery spree, I felt like a new human being. The circus in my mind was still in town, but at least I had met the performers, learned a few acts. And they couldn't terrorize me to the extent they were able to when I wasn't familiar with them. In the following chapters, I'd focus on taming those acts. Calming the jittery acrobat and silencing (or at least shushing) the inner critic clown. But none of it would have unfolded if not for that initial pulling back of the curtain to see who was behind the performance. Knowing that the "circus" can be treated with curiosity and fun is my daily reminder that this chaos is not me; it's just one facet of my mental terrain. That revelation alone turns dread into fascination. And maybe a bit of joy. Well now that I get the spectacle, now I need to learn how to share the stage with it. Chapter 6, "Embracing the Struggle," explores what it takes to live with these performances, turning the messy magic into an avenue for growth, resilience and, ultimately, even deeper self-compassion.

Chapter 6: Embracing the Struggle

We chant 'no pain, no gain,' but the real victory comes when you can joke about the bruises, because if you're laughing, you're still in the fight.

Gym-goers have a saying, "No pain, no gain!" somehow piercing the din of clanking barbells. Trainers shout it, gym buddies echo it, and lathered neophytes grab their sore muscles and pray it's true. The idea has morphed into some kind of catchall philosophy, insinuating that real progress, in terms of fitness, career or personal growth, comes with a certain dose of suffering, as if we're on a collective treadmill of misery. Yet is "no pain, no gain" a universal theorem for betterment, or a well-meaning adage evolved into self-flagellating dogma? How much pain is good for us, though, and how do we differentiate productive struggle from pointless suffering?

This chapter is an opportunity to flex our mental muscles exploring the challenge in finding the balance of effort versus growth. We'll explore the precise truth of pain having to lead to gain in terms of physical training, delve into social science experiments that show how the difficulty of an effort leads us to attribute greater value to it and ponder the insights of modern psychology around "grit" and the "growth mindset." Along the way, expect some comic references, you can't, after all, hate the tedious struggle of a sweaty, clumsy new skill, without hating the whole experience, in which case, what's the point? By the end, you'll understand that "embracing the struggle" isn't so much about glorifying pain as it is about acknowledging that some discomfort, if applied correctly, can make us soar to new heights.

The Literal Interpretation of "No Pain, No Gain"

On a strictly biological basis, the saying "no pain, no gain" contains a grain of truth in strength training. Schoenfeld (2010) indicates that resistance exercise can create microdamage in muscle fibers, stimulating various anabolic pathways during recovery. Over time, these processes increase fiber size, confirming the basic tenet that "a small amount of harm" signals adaptation and growth. This scientific rationale underpins the colloquial maxim "no pain, no gain," so long as the "pain" is moderate and does not cross into injury territory. The body repairs those tiny injuries by laying down more, thicker fibers and building muscle. Without that small amount of harm, your body does not have the signal to change, meaning you remain on the same basis. This principle, called muscle hypertrophy, reinforces the idea that genuine growth usually comes at the cost of some pain.

There's a difference, of course, between the right amount of pain, mild soreness, or an effort that's challenging but not overwhelming, and excess (which leads to actual injury, or a chronic strain). Lift too much or fail to rest, and it's possible to tear a muscle, in a way that promises all pain, no gain. Metaphorically, however, it's a lovely metaphor: measured hardship catalyzes adaptation; extreme hardship breaks us.

Psychologists call this "stress inoculation," referring to the concept of exposure to manageable stressors building resilience, similar to how a vaccine introduces a weakened version of a virus, allowing your immune system to learn to combat the real thing (Meichenbaum, 1988). Without undergoing any difficulty, you have no need to develop new coping skills. But being too challenged can lead to burnout. The best balance is enough discomfort that adaptation is warranted, not so much that you're flattened."

We even have research suggesting that humans are sometimes effort-seekers. So while we try to avoid unnecessary stress, there's evidence in cognitive science that paradoxically, we assign more value to the outcomes for which we've expended more effort (Inzlicht, et. al, 2018). It's like wanting that "I earned this" feeling, not merely a handout. If you've ever devoted hours to jigsaw puzzling incomprehensible do-it-yourself furniture into place, then grimly felt a sense of pride, "This is the most fabulous shelf, even if it leans left!", you've tasted that effect. The effort put in can add subjective value to an achievement.

Sweat Equity: Effort Justification in Everyday Life

A classic social psychology study found that "pain," or at least some discomfort, enhances our bond to a group (Aronson & Mills, 1959). In the experiment, college-age women volunteered to join a discussion group but had to undergo an "embarrassment test" to get into it, with some reading aloud sexually explicit material and others undergoing a mild or no initiation. Afterward, they all could hear the same monotonous reasoning. The troublesome result: The women who went through the more degrading initiation rated the discussion (still boring!) as more fun and more rewarding to read. This phenomenon, known as "effort justification," is surprisingly resilient.

We witness it with institutions with difficult admission procedures. Grueling pledge weeks for fraternities or sororities create incredibly loyal members, in part because the suffering "proves" the group is special. Or consider backpacking into a gorgeous, remote valley. If you've spent days caring your way over steep terrain, battling bug bites and dwindling water supplies, you may find the valley more stunning than you would have if you'd simply driven to an overlook. Humans, it seems, tend to justify or inflate the worth of anything they have labored for.

Of course, this can go sideways into irrational territory, some groups or pursuits simply are not worthy, no matter how much they hurt to pursue. But sometimes putting in sweat equity really does create a deeper appreciation and reward. "Satisfaction lies in the effort, not in the attainment; full effort is full victory," Gandhi is said to have remarked. Because this might help explain why completing a marathon on which you limped to the finish line is much more memorable than breezing through a 5K that barely broke a sweat. Striving through struggle, even acute pain, turns your achievement (and long-distance running very much count as an achievement) from an idle pastime into a personal triumph.

Using Discomfort as a tool

In real life "no pain, no gain" serves us well so long as we think of "pain" as a struggle with a goal in mind. When you're learning a new instrument, your fingers are probably sore at first' guitar calluses don't develop overnight' but that slight discomfort is the cost of getting better. But you wouldn't go out of your way to damage your fingers to the point of absurdity, thinking that suffering begets excellence. Likewise, for Christians, 100-hour weeks could also entail "pain" of a sort, but the burnout and failing health that result create a toxic net sum.

That's where the real magic happens' picking the frontiers on either side of the optimal difficulty zone. The Zone of Proximal Development, as psychologists call it, is about tasks or skills just beyond your reach that challenge you to stretch, but not so far that you fall apart (Vygotsky, 1978). It's like gradually increasing your exercise in sports, not jumping from sleep to a marathon. In academics, it's about taking a challenging class that broadens your knowledge, not overwhelms you with unmanageable workloads. This zone, with its balance of tension and stress, ensures that you're always in a state of manageable challenge, giving you the confidence to push your limits.

A thought exercise: Maria wants to pursue her first novel. She has never written anything longer than a short essay. If she promises herself a challenging but achievable daily word count, let's say 1,000 words, she may experience emotional pain, frustration and self-doubt ("What if it's terrible?"), but by persevering, she develops discipline. After weeks or months, she's got a messy first draft. What if Maria had said, "If it's meant to be, it should come naturally," and walked away at the first sign of struggle? She would be stuck without a manuscript. Here, the short-term discomfort of making herself write won over inertia and released a sense of achievement.

Grit and the Growth Mindset

The term "grit" is a modern psychological concept that refers to one's perseverance and quest for long-term goals (Duckworth, 2016). Angela Duckworth, the psychologist who popularized the term, found that "gritty" people often beat out people with higher I.Q. or talent but less grit. They just don't give up when the going gets tough. They embrace adversity, presumably adopting a "no pain, no gain" mentality that considers friction a steppingstone and not a stop sign.

Duckworth's work also intersects with growth mindset. This is a phrase to capture the belief that abilities can be fostered with effort (Dweck, 2006). A growth mindset considers struggle and mistakes to be typical steps in the learning process' pain is progress. And if you bomb a test, you might take it as useful feedback: "I need to practice more of these kinds of problems." In contrast, a fixed mindset would say, "I bombed because I'm just not good at math. The latter perspective stymies further exertion, since pain or failure registers as proof of inherent inability, rather than a signal that you're expanding beyond your comfort zone.

That has real-world consequences. Such students are more likely to select complex tasks, recover from failure, and eventually learn skills (Dweck, 2006). Athletes who accept that every new workout should challenge them 'without promising instant reward, tend to advance faster. In daily life, if you're faced with a specific challenging project at work, we're more resilient if you see this as an opportunity to learn new skills, whereas seeing something challenging as evidence you're simply "not cut out for this" leads to stagnation.

And of course, humans are also prone to value things more when we've struggled for them. Psychologists refer to it as the "IKEA effect" (Norton et al., 2012), after our tendency to overestimate the value of furniture we assemble ourselves, no matter how much it wobbles. The time and slight pain we spend figuring out nonsensical instructions make the product more precious. It can apply to most parts of life: from raising kids (so much lost sleep, but so much love) to making a complicated meal from scratch (you'll treasure every bite even more than if it was delivered in a microwave tray).

Meanwhile, some Eastern philosophies point out that struggle can sharpen priorities and fortify discipline. We have more systematic frameworks around that idea now: stress inoculation, effort justification, growth mindset, etc. All converge on the principle that powering through well-chosen difficulties leads to growth.

But the temptation is always to fetishize suffering for its own sake. If you're torturing yourself simply to "prove toughness," you may pay in injuries or bitterness. The true secret is that all-important purposeful struggle, which could look like practicing an instrument, learning a language, honing a skill or training your body, where the discomfort or challenge directly augments the evolutionary process.

When Pain Goes Too Far

Not all pain yields gain. In sports, overtraining can cause injuries that will bench you for months. Aspirations to overperform academically or professionally can quickly lead to burnout, at which point you are too fatigued to be adequately productive, ultimately losing more than you accrue in the long term (Maslach et al., 2001). Even in a psychological sense, forcing yourself too much can bring about mental health crises. If you're sleep-deprived, for example, your attempts to study more or practice more may yield diminishing returns and just end up breaking down.

One classic example in psychology is the Yerkes-Dodson law: performance increases with physiological or mental (e.g., stress) arousal up to a point, and then it decreases with higher arousal levels than optimal (Yerkes & Dodson, 1908). That's why a small dose of adrenaline before giving a public speech might narrow your focus, but a full-fledged panic attack can sabotage your delivery. In the same way, moderate struggle promotes engagement, though far too difficult a challenge may lead you to either give up or falter under stress.

Real-World Struggle: Case Studies

Let's imagine two fictional people, both facing a major challenge:

Alex, bored in their repetitive 9-to-5, wants a way out and decides they will learn to code. The first weeks are hell: mistakes in code that yield nothing, jargon that might as well be Martian. Alex's eyes are sore from late-night study, encouragement wanes. But Alex presses on, fueled by online tutorials, small victories (finally getting a simple program to run) and a growth mindset that each error is a clue, not a death sentence. Eventually, through months of this painful learning curve, Alex builds a demo project, gets the attention of a startup, and scores an entry-level developer role. Alex would never have gained the skill set without the original pain, those all-nighters, debugging disasters, self-doubt.

Brenda wants to run a marathon, but she's never jogged more than a mile. Her early training sessions are humbling shin splints, gasped breaths, and the mortifying discovery that she can't keep up with even casual runners. A friend suggests taking baby steps' perhaps the first goal is a 5K, next a half-marathon. Brenda suffers aches and pains, spends money on better shoes, and carefully rests between runs to keep from getting hurt. She completes her first half-marathon after months. Later, she tries the full 26.2 miles. It's a strenuous race, but crossing that finish line, tears in her eyes, she feels a huge sense of accomplishment. That discomfort was all too real, but it drove her to do something that was unthinkable a year before.

In either case, it's not the pain alone that yields results. Its pain and purposeful work, redirected struggle, with the acknowledgment that recovery and gradual progress count. It's the struggle that breeds not just the external (coding job, marathon medal) but the internal (confidence, discipline, a feeling of expanded possibility).

Balancing Effort with Rest

One aspect that gets overlooked is rest and recovery. Muscles, be they physical or metaphorical, grow in rest periods, after they've been challenged. Which is why bodybuilders preach the benefit of rest days and a sufficient intake of protein. In much the same way the brain consolidates learning in sleep and breaks, (Mednick & Ehrman, 2006). Too many of us forget that working ourselves to the bone might erode performance. You are not weak for needing downtime. You're just in concert with how bodies and minds really adapt.

And this principle holds even for if not emotional or mental challenges. If you continue to push yourself too hard to cope with every occupier 'compoundly' heaping rise tasks without giving your mind a chance to catch up' you may notice a decline in creativity, motivation, or even body health. The philosophy of "no pain, no gain" needs to be tempered with "no rest, no progress."

The saying "no pain, no gain" resonates in part because it's a concise awareness-raising statement about the good kind of suffering: mild difficulty can serve as the basis for genuine progress. We see it in muscles in the most literal sense: microtears that recover even stronger. We experience it in social experiments such as Aronson and Mills (1959), where paying a painful price has people holding something in higher esteem. We observe it in grit and growth mindset research (Duckworth, 2016; Dweck, 2006) demonstrating that sticking-to-it despite adversity often trumps raw talent.

Yet we must avoid extremes. Not all pain is helpful. Chronic burnout, or physical injuries, illustrate that suffering without a limit can erode the very benefits we are striving for. We also risk glorifying pain for pain's sake, losing sight of its utility as a driver of adaptation, not a tool for self-blindsiding.

In real life, the sweet spot is when we choose things that are just outside our comfort zone, lean into the discomfort, and recover adequately. Those who have gone through trial and tribulation often say that what they've been through showed them strengths they never knew existed or taught them things that would only come through failure and adversity rather than success. But this is the crux of "embracing the struggle" the acceptance of constructive discomfort, not the pursuit of futile agony.

Key Takeaways

- Effort and discomfort are often prerequisites for growth. Our bodies and minds adapt to challenges (muscles strengthen after strain; skills improve after difficult practice). No challenge means no improvement.
- We value what we earn. Through effort justification, people tend to love outcomes they worked hard for more than easy wins. The satisfaction from achievement is heightened by the knowledge of struggles overcome.
- Grit matters. Perseverance in the face of difficulty (a "no pain, no gain" attitude) is linked to higher odds of success in many domains. Sticking with challenges when others quit is a competitive advantage.
- Not all pain is productive. The goal is purposeful pain – the kind that signals growth. Too much pain (overtraining, burnout) is harmful. Balance effort with recovery. Think "no challenge, no gain" – one must be pushed outside the comfort zone but not pushed off a cliff.
- Mindset is key. Embracing challenges as opportunities (growth mindset) makes the inevitable pains of learning feel worthwhile, not something to be avoided at all costs. Short-term discomfort leads to long-term capability.

"No pain, no gain" is a reminder that deliberate effort, and discomfort can be a catalyst for real growth. We are not to seek pain indiscriminately or romanticize suffering for the sake of suffering, but when we are challenged, and when we seek challenges that connect us with our string of wins. Whether it's physical training, learning a new skill, working on something personal that we need to accomplish, we realize and tap into our own resilience and deeper reserve of discipline.

In the Chapter 7, "Don't Judge a Book By Its Cover", we'll turn the lens from our internal battles to our external judgment of others. Just as extreme outliers may expand the limits of our personal growth, becoming able to look past appearances may deepen our connections with the world around us. It's a different kind of challenge, one that calls for empathy rather than endurance, and curiosity rather than complacency. Let's see how which looking beyond the "cover" could lead to new books or avenues of understanding and acceptance being opened.

Chapter 7: Don't Judge a Book by Its Cover

If the cover of books were the only thing to consider, I think we would have read the whole world by now. Wouldn't we?

In a viral 2009 moment, a modest, middle-aged woman named Susan Boyle walked onstage on Britain's Got Talent (Leyland, 2009). She handled herself somewhat shyly, wearing a basic dress, and did not fit the glittery picture many envisioned of a talent show star. Audience members laughed freely, and the judges hardly hid their contempt. She then started singing, and in a few seconds the whole audience went from jeers to thunderous acclaim. Boyle's performance broke the cynical presumption that her frightened, understated look matched poor aptitude. Many people stated, we messed up by condemning her on sight. Dr. Brooks (2009) considered how rapidly the audience came to see its bias once the truth of her voice surfaced. That lightning-fast reversal summed up a recurrent lesson: human people often misjudge based on superficial appearances, only to be catastrophically, or pleasantly, wrong.

Snap Decisions and Their Motives

Evolutionary thinkers suggest that people make hasty decisions since quick decisions once helped survival (Haselton & Buss, 2000). When our forebears came upon an unidentified person in the wild, they had to act fast to determine if that person was friend or enemy or risk a fatal result. Modern psychologists such as Todorov et. al. (2005) contend that this ancient mechanism still runs: we create perceptions of competence or trustworthiness from a face in a fraction of a second. Of course, the issue is that modern life hardly depends on indications from primordial danger. The person we are measuring up could be a job candidate in mismatched socks, an uncomfortable coworker, or (yes) a possible star with a quiet manner. Sometimes our old survival response results in faulty conclusions since we make decisions on unquestioned superficial signs.

The way the brain insists on quick paths that make sense on a savanna but occasionally betrays us in an audition hall strikes me as curiously funny. Alternatively, a face we label "unfriendly" could just reflect someone's distracted thinking about a missing mortgage payment or the next week's test. As Todorov et al. (2005) demonstrated, we attach broad generalizations, like "They look competent! "to quick peeks." That could have kept cavemen free from a sabretooth or hostile tribe, but it might compromise us in a well-lit conference room or on a reality TV platform.

The Halo Effect

The "halo effect," is a major bias that leads to these quick judgments Thorndike (1920). This happens when one positive trait, like being beautiful or wearing stylish clothes, affects how we see other positive traits, like being smart or kind. We think to ourselves, "Since she's pretty, she must also be smart, organized, and genuinely caring." On the other hand, if someone's "cover" is crazy, messy, or boring, we might think they are less smart or moral.

The funny side shows itself when we think about how often clever looks fool us. Consider how a well-dressed con artist, radiating confidence, may fool gullible people, land loans, or pass employment interviews. Frank Abagnale, who told his adventures in Catch Me If You Can, notably passed for doctors and pilots by dressing in the correct outfit and manner (Abagnale & Redding, 2000). He made great use of the halo effect: dressing in the right "cover" instantly established credibility. A true genius might show up in worn-out sweatpants at the same time, which we would discount. The mind essentially says, "Great cover, must be a great book", or "Not so great cover, probably useless content."

We could laugh at how ridiculous that is, but it's no joke when the consequences shape hiring decisions, political votes, or daily social acceptance. Todorov et al. (2005) noted that these facial-based judgments are not just minor quirks; they can predict things like election outcomes if voters see a politician's face and perceive "competence," or "weakness." When they mislead us, even funny illusions have major consequences.

Job interviews, dating apps, and missing geniuses

Like job interviews, we observe cover-based bias in everyday settings. According to Hamermesh and Biddle (1994), physically beautiful people typically make more money, sometimes 10–15% more than similarly capable colleagues. The theory is that colleagues and companies automatically react better to the "good cover" of a pleasing countenance. One can find a comparable function in height. Taller male candidates are generally seen as more "leader-like," according to Hamermesh and Parker (2005), even in the absence of actual data showing they really lead better. Thinking about how these surface signals eclipse more fundamental qualities like creativity, empathy, or problem-solving ability is both funny and sad.

Dating applications might often show reckless quick judgments gone crazy. People slide left or right depending on a few pictures. Though the latter might have a heart of gold or an unrivaled sense of humor, even in offline dating a sharp dresser might catch curiosity more easily than someone wearing mismatched socks. Once a friend complained that she had a date bail mid-evening just because she had chosen a low-key dress, and her hair was somewhat twisted. She said that if she had worn a business-casual jacket, the date might have stayed with her to find her sharp discussion. Rather, the date appraised a "messy cover," concluded "messy person," and missed out.

Sneakier is how we could discount possible geniuses or inventors who don't seem "professional." Steve Jobs, known for his jeans and turtleneck, was famously messy in early Atari days, eating people's ears off about radical computing concepts. Perhaps Jobs would have been swiftly terminated if the manager had insisted on a suit-and-tie formality, therefore hindering Apple's revolution. Imagine a modern-day Einstein walking into a business environment with messy hair and a dirty sweater and being turned away by a suspicious guard, that would be funny.

Cover-Based Stereotypes

Until we understand that snap decisions based on covers, clothing, ethnicity, gender, even a name, can support systematic injustices, it's all fun and games. In a well-known field experiment on labor market discrimination, Bertrand and Mullainathan (2004) found that identical resumes with "white-sounding" names, like Emily or Greg, received 50% more responses than those with "African American-sounding" names, like Lakisha or Jamal. This involves evaluating the "book," or application, using a flimsy criterion that fuels prejudice. People are rejected positions for which they are qualified merely because HR managers' implicit (or conscious) bias says, "That name signals a not-so-good cover." This loses the humorous aspect.

In casual social situations, prejudice can cause us to avoid those from another culture or who dress differently. We create homogeneous buddy circles over time that lose opportunities to learn from many points of view. According to polls like one by Reuters/Ipsos (2013), about 40% of White Americans have few or no non-White friends. Partly that's about geographical separation, but also partly about an inability to interact with people we consider to be "unfamiliar." We can be missing great friendships just because we assume the "cover" denotes we have nothing in common.

When law enforcement or vigilantes encounter shallow assessments, the outcome may be fatal. If an observer decides "cover = threat," ignoring the reality of an unarmed kid simply walking home, disaster can follow. The 2012 shooting of Black teenager Trayvon Martin, wearing a hoodie, became typical of how dangerous it is to rely on assumptions about someone "looks suspicious." The proverb "Don't judge a book by its cover" thus leaps from gently moral advice to urgent, life-saving wisdom: we must challenge our instincts before acting on them as though they were truths.

How Cooperatively Deceive in Media and Marketing

We do it with everything from restaurants to books, not simply persons we misunderstand by appearances. Perhaps you pass by a hole-in-the- wall restaurant due of its run-down façade only to find later that it offers the best pho or tacos for the area. On the other hand, once you sample its pricey, average cuisine, a slick, high-end bistro may not be impressive. As the saying goes, "all that glitters is not gold." The humorous point of view is that whole marketing plans center on this phenomenon, product designers know people react strongly to surface cues. While a wonderfully designed cover could propel a weak novel to best-seller status until word-of-mouth discloses the reality, a poorly designed book cover might destroy a great manuscript.

I remember once missing a book with a boring cover that seemed done in Microsoft Paint. You must read it, a buddy argued, and I surrendered and found an amazing story. Had I not listened, I would have missed out simply because the "cover" was an aesthetic failure. For the same reason, we humans cannot help but evaluate the packaging, the entertainment business spends significantly in dazzling trailers, billboard graphics, and celebrity sponsorships.

Techniques for Beyond the Cover Look-ahead

Given our inclination to these delusions, how might we slow down? I like to follow what I'll call the "cover test." The moment I find myself instantaneously fascinated or contemptuous of someone, I ask: "Am I responding mostly to an outward cue, clothing, accent, posture, or name? And what if the reality is different? If possible, I could have them converse. If it's anything like a book or a new brand of cereal, I might search more closely through reviews or sample a page or two.

Structured or "blind" procedures help if you can assess individuals, say in employment or admittance contexts. Many orchestras started employing blind auditions, musicians perform behind a screen, and Goldin and Rouse (2000) found that this resulted in higher hiring of female musicians. That's literally reading the "book" by its contents, its sound, rather than the performer's gender. To minimize prejudices about race, gender, or age, some employers are using anonymized resumes and deleting names or images.

We can individually also question the "halo effect" (Thorndike, 1920). Should we find ourselves too taken in by someone's polished appearance or voice, we wonder, "Do I have proof this person is really talented or friendly? Conversely, if someone's disheveled appearance irritates us, can we identify anything about their substance to challenge our presumptions? Though first forced, this is like training ourselves to think, "Wait, maybe that hole-in- the wall restaurant is a hidden gem," or "maybe that quiet colleague in sneakers is actually a coding wizard."

At last, comic self-awareness can be useful. Often, I find myself drawn to flimsy objects, like a friend walking over an introduction or someone sporting name-brand shoes. The second I perceive the irony, I can back off and say, "All right, let's see some real data." I remind myself, "Silly me, I'm letting a shoe brand impress me or a stutter deter me."

Moment as a Global Wake-Up Call: Susan Boyle

The whole Britain's Got Talent theatre burst in ovation after Susan Boyle ended her performance of "I Dreamed a Dream (Britain's Got Talent, 2009). Originally very dismissively, Judge Simon Cowell freely said it was the biggest surprise he had come across. Psychologist Robert Brooks (2009) reported that her performance went viral online fast, drawing millions of viewers to a clip that succinctly declared, "We all got it wrong. We assessed her using flimsy criteria.

Many viewers felt both ashamed of their early pessimism and delighted by her win at the same time since that reversal was so unexpected. Comedically, it was a gotcha moment: everyone gets manipulated by their own prejudice. On social media, analysts owned up to having laughed or felt sorry for her, never expecting brilliance. She turned the whole script inside a few seconds. That makes it relevant as a timeless warning story.

I remember a buddy who, upon seeing Susan Boyle's audition, commented, "I can't believe I was part of that crowd in spirit, assuming she'd fail." He understood how readily our brains mix external appearance with underlying talent. The funny punch is how easy it was for her to disprove everyone. She just had to open her mouth and sing for around one minute. That quick disintegration of illusions tells us that next time we see a similarly "unassuming" figure, we can check the temptation to snickle and wait to see whether there is concealed genius.

Stopping Before Cover Closing

While it's a reflex, judging a book by its cover might cost us. The "packaging" didn't appeal to us, thus we might pass on a great friendship, a brilliant hire, or a mouthwatering dinner. On the other hand, we might overstate a polished charmer without substance. The first step in correcting the mistake is realizing how quickly we create shallow perceptions (Todorov et al., 2005) and how often they mislead us.

The smart course is to slow down, compile actual data, give individuals or experiences a fair go. The next time you're ready to dismiss someone who looks awkward or plain or to idolize someone who's got all the superficial signs of "success," consider the comic possibility that you could be hilariously off-track. It does not mean ignoring real red flags.

Key Takeaways

- First impressions can mislead. We all make snap judgments based on looks (face, clothing, demeanor), but these are often inaccurate. Spectacular talents or qualities may hide behind ordinary exteriors (e.g., Susan Boyle's case), and conversely, a polished appearance can mask incompetence or ill intent.
- Biases in favor of appearance are real. Attractive or well-presented individuals tend to be judged more favorably in hiring, social settings, etc., despite no inherent link to ability. This leads to unfair advantages and missed opportunities to recognize true merit.
- Surface traits ≠ content. Stereotypes based on race, attire, accent, etc., can be very misleading (as shown in studies like the résumé name experiment). Many important qualities – intelligence, kindness, integrity – are not accurately measurable from appearance alone.
- Take time to gather evidence. To avoid misjudging, consciously pause and get to know the person or situation better. Use blind or content-focused evaluations when possible. Recognize when you might be falling for the "halo effect" or other biases.

- Classic wisdom holds true: "All that glitters is not gold" and "Appearances are deceiving." True value often lies beneath the surface. Whether evaluating people, products, or opportunities, dig deeper than face value. In doing so, you'll make fairer decisions and discover gems that others might overlook.

And in the end, judge slowly and kindly. Whether it's a silent colleague hiding exceptional talent, a worn paper back on the shelf concealing literary gold, or a new friend whose quirks may be their best asset. True worth may lie just beneath the surface. By forcing ourselves to look deeper and stay open-minded, we give ourselves the gift of discovery and remind one another that substance trumps packaging a mile.

To judge a person or a situation by appearances is a dangerous business. Our first clips of an impression might hide a deep talent; your knee-jerk reaction might expose your hidden bias. But not all cover is on the outside. Often, the most insidious "cover" is the face we put on when we're feeling encumbered by internal conflict. In Chapter 8 "Climbing Out of Depression", we will transition from outer illusions to the deafening, ghastly silence that often you bring inside due to numbing heaviness. We'll dig into the small steps, glimmers of hope, and even moments of joy that can help brighten the darkest corners of the mind. It's like going from a world of quick judgments to a closer examination of how we are judging ourselves when life feels gray, and how we may find enough light, or braveness to climb up.".

Chapter 8: Climbing Out of Depression

Even the darkest of clouds eventually run out of rain.

Where anxiety resembled a runaway circus, the panting ringmaster hurling panic-pot instead of doom-time bulletins, depression was its antithesis: a torpid, grimly expanding plunge into quicksand. Anxiety, as far as I could tell, in me, had a wired, restless energy: the wanting to do something, anything, to get away from dread. Depression, though, came as a dark hush, an emptying of motivation or spark, a hollow heaviness that pressed me down. After spending months learning how to alleviate panic and worry, I found myself faced with a new foe hiding beneath those emotions: a slump of low mood and disinterest that caught me off guard. Psychologist Jamison (1995), known for her work on mood disorders, observes that anxiety and depression frequently coexist, with one emerging after the other recedes. My experience verified this idea: as my nervous storms became more controllable, a stronger wave of despair set in.

An Unexpected Shift: From Anxiety to Numbness

A few months into therapy, I had felt I was on a decent path: fewer panic attacks, better sleep and even some laughs with friends. Then I noticed a deep fatigue that no amount of normal rest could alleviate. I would wake up at a decent hour, then fall back into bed until noon. Things I used to enjoy, writing, painting, having coffee with friends, seemed not just unattractive but almost futile. How, as Beck (1976) explains, clinical depression can rob activities of their usual pleasure and how, the joke being on this tortured mind, no matter how many hours I slept there would remain an ache of tiredness in my bones.

When I shared this new malaise with Dr. Nguyen, she reframed it: "This could have been lingering underneath anxiety from the very beginning," Dr. Nguyen pointed out, "or it could be a result of coming down off the drug of months of constant stress." Such an observation fits with what (Casacalenda et al., 2002) refer to as "comorbid presentations," wherein treating one disorder (like panic) only partially reveals another one (like depression). For me, the great tragicomic joke was that after experiencing a flicker of triumph over anxiety, I came to realize I had accidentally walked in on a denser, slugger beast that apparently wanted its own strategy guide.

The Quiet Manifestations of Depression

Depression isn't always the usual picture of crying uncontrollably or listening to sad music. Most of the time, it's a numb nothingness or not being able to feel anything at all. The National Institute of Mental Health (NIMH, 2018) says that for many people, depression is mainly marked by a severe loss of interest (anhedonia) and extreme tiredness, which makes small chores seem very difficult. That was a great description of me. Some weekends I would sleep until noon and then wake up to mindlessly scroll through my phone and maybe start a load of laundry before giving up and going back to sleep. I wasn't exactly crying or feeling hopeless; I was simply numb.

For me, it was a cruel catch-22. Depression can also create the sensation of learned helplessness: a belief that nothing one does really matters (Seligman, 1975). That can make exactly the activities that might help — socializing, exercising, pursuing hobbies — seem impossible, thanks to low energy or motivation. A trusted professional I spoke with called it the "friction of depression," the urge to force yourself forward even though every gesture feels like it's being dragged through molasses.

Climbing Out: A Slow, Uneven Process

Depression often demands a gentler, more patient approach than anxiety—while grounding techniques or laughter can sometimes soothe anxiety in the moment, they don't necessarily ignite the lost energy and hope characteristic of depression. I quickly discovered that applying "super-charged anxiety solutions" to depression was ineffective; depression isn't about taming overactive alarms so much as rekindling any spark of vitality. In line with Parker, Roy, and Eyers's (2003) view that therapy for depression benefits from a deliberately paced and individualized strategy, recovery often unfolds in small, incremental steps rather than in sweeping leaps.

On this slow walk, I likened myself to walking through mud: every step a labor, no immediate sense of triumph, but critical all the same. Dr. Nguyen suggested behavioral activation, a technique developed by Jacobson, Martell and Dimidjian (2001) that interrupts the cycle of avoidance by scheduling small, pleasurable or purposeful tasks, even if I was not motivated to do so. At first, it felt forced. One day, I opened my watercolor palette and set a timer for 10 minutes, just to do aimless watercolors. I wasn't about to paint a masterpiece, but for that stretch, I concentrated on pigment instead of my mental fog. It may sound humorous to call it progress, but as Dr. Nguyen noted, "Any movement fights depression's inertia."

Small Steps on a Slippery Slope

Depression deflates energy so thoroughly that mundane tasks, responding to texts, making breakfast, seem monumental. For example, Burns (1989) emphasizes that depressed cognition is failure-magnifying and success-disqualifying, fostering a sense of futility. My strategy evolved into mini goals: "Stand on the porch for five minutes of fresh air," "Text one friend," or "Cook one meal with vegetables." Tiny though this may sound, each small success added a grain to its momentum.

A friend named Maria once made me go to brunch. I had gone half-reluctant, and we ended up laughing at an unpremeditated joke. That tiny flicker of real laughter surprised me; I remembered that, for a second, I wasn't numb. According to Hammen (2018), social support may be a buffer against depression, in part by countering isolation and self-critical thinking. My comedic reflection? Depression's command had been "Stay in bed; you're too exhausted," but brunch gave me, ironically, a momentary semblance of normalcy.

Routines also helped. I imposed on myself a regular wake time, a brief morning walk and a going-to-bed routine. While doing so felt like a medicated, forced march, a mere tenet of practice, Brown et al., (2014) suggest that proper sleep and gentle daily mobilization can help alleviate neurotransmitter dysregulation associated with mood.

Gratitude and the Slow Thaw

I also started a gratitude practice, which mildly improve mood by focusing on positive aspects of daily life (Seligman et al., 2005). I learned to write things like, "I'm grateful I found clean socks." It felt ridiculous, like I was grasping for anything upbeat. But as each little taste of gratitude, like "I appreciate the friendliest wave from the neighbor" or "My coffee was pretty good", made its way to the page, it infused tiny pinpricks of light into a gray mental canvas. In the ensuing weeks, these repeated acknowledgments held me together, a reminder that life wasn't all darkness, despite what depression would have had me believe.

Of course, severe depression or any trace of self-harm requires professional assistance. Therapy, or sometimes medication, or both, can be lifesaving for major depressive episodes (American Psychiatric Association, 2020). Dr. Nguyen and I, made a safety plan: if I ever felt like I was nearing the edge, I had a list of contacts, including a crisis line, along with specific steps like "Play an uplifting song," "Look at comforting photos," or "Text a friend saying, 'I'm not okay.'" The funny part is how earnest and even life-saving that plan was, but it might include instructions as detailed as "Watch your favorite goofy YouTube cat video." Occasionally a sense of humor is part of the safety net.

Progress, Not Perfection

The climb out of depression is seldom a neat upward incline. In a 1976 paper, Beck argues that people might experience temporary benefits, followed by deterioration, then re-improvement. The frustration sets in when you've had a decent run, maybe a few days of productive energy, and then you crash again. Early on I called it "backsliding," but Dr. Nguyen reframed it as normal fluctuation. She explained that short blips don't override the overall upward trend, likening it to the stock market: what looks like day-to-day volatility can obscure a long-term rise.

I remember one week thinking I'd made real progress, successfully completing chores and attending a friend's birthday, and the next weekend barely moving from my couch. The ironic humor is that I was "feeling better," but also still "feeling awful," two states that can mesh into something of a collage. Over time I learned to accept that depression lifts in starts and stops. We learn patience, something I, with an anxious mind that craved quick fixes, needed to be taught.

Empathy Gained and My Changed Perspective

One surprising result was how my own depression deepened my empathy for others who suffer. I would think to myself, "Why can't they just get up and do something?" or "Maybe they're lazy." But once I had sunk into that bog myself, I understood what a strong gravitational pull it can exert. I once rolled out my eyes at the phrase "can't get out of bed" the same way I'd roll them at "could care less", a little frustrated, but mostly amused. That was before it was my life.

When I started to come out of the worst phases, I felt softer toward people's limits. If a friend said, "I can't handle going out tonight," I no longer joked, "Oh, come on, be social." Instead, I would reply, "I understand. Let's do something low-key or reschedule." This change in perspective, ironically, was a gift Depression left behind. I wouldn't wish the condition on anyone, but the empathy it encourages can be a silver lining (Jamison, 1995).

The Humor in Hopelessness

If I found myself pinned down by negative thoughts, "Everything is meaningless," "I'll never get better", I would occasionally picture the voice of a narrator flamboyantly announcing: "And now, starring in the low-energy gloom spectacular, we have Felicity!" It wasn't a cure, but it provided me with a moment of levity or perspective. Beck and Emery (1985) suggest that getting out of your own catastrophic monologue can moderately liberate you from the vise grip of depression.

Sometimes I'd overhear my own comedic self-deprecation: "So I'm worthless and my cat hates me? That's quite the storyline." That small distance allowed me to look at how outrageous some depressed thoughts were. For comedy's sake, my cat, who would ironically be the only living creature thrilled to see me passed out on the couch all day for extra cuddles, was slowly getting away from the chewing because he worked up an appetite munching (cleaning) up a substance's spillage. This soft humor wasn't a way to trivialize real pain; it was a wedge, keeping me slightly apart from abject despair.

Therapeutic, Pharmacological and Lifestyle Effects

Many need some sort of professional intervention in moderate or severe cases. I was the sort of person who found therapy essential. Medication can also be important, though I didn't end up taking antidepressants. Selective Serotonin Reuptake Inhibitors (SSRIs) the class of drugs made famous for correcting a specific imbalance of neurotransmitters in the brain (NIMH, 2018), can bring unwanted symptoms associated with depression down to a significantly more manageable level for some individuals. The comedic stigma around pills, such as the idea of them as "cheater's solutions", can make people refrain from getting help. But suppose Dr. Nguyen would say, "If you need them, it's no different than taking medication for diabetes or high blood pressure." That idea beats the short-circuiting delusions about "toughing it out."

Lifestyle changes, such as exercise, nutrition, or mindfulness, can also help (just know, vegan or non-vegan, organic or nonorganic it's your good business). Even low-level physical activity is linked to improved mood, 15-minute walks a day, for example (Dimidjian et. al., 2014). The funny perspective is how ridiculous it was to congratulate "I walked around the block!" as if it was a marathon. But to a depressed mind, this can feel like climbing Everest. So, yes, I self-administered a mental high-five for these small wins.

Trying New Tools: Mindfulness and Self-Compassion

In parallel with behavioral activation, Dr. Nguyen introduced me to mindfulness, reminiscent of Kabat-Zinn's (1990) approach: observe thoughts and feelings without immediate reaction or judgment. Initially, it seemed too gentle to battle the heaviness. But ironically, noticing "I'm feeling numb, and that's okay" sometimes diffused the frustration of wanting numbness to vanish. The humor can be to picture my negative thoughts as leaves floating past on a stream: "Oh, look, there's the 'I'm worthless' leaf. Bye-bye." Each time I tried this, I realized I didn't have to cling to those thoughts or let them define me.

Self-compassion, a related concept highlighted by Neff (2011), was another big shift. In depression, we often add insult to injury by berating ourselves for feeling low: "Ugh, I'm so weak. Why can't I function like normal people?" Replacing that with kindness, "I'm struggling, and that's not my fault. I can do little steps today.", opened a gentler, more supportive internal monologue. The comedic angle is that it was easier for me to show compassion to a friend's sadness but not my own. Realizing that double standard was comedic enough to push me to treat myself like I'd treat a loved one: with understanding and encouragement rather than scorn.

The Emergence of Hope

Slowly, these interventions of different kinds, small steps, therapy, some mild exercise, routine, humor, coalesced into some upward trend. One day, I suddenly thought, "I want to cook and eat one of my favorite recipes! One night, I suddenly called a friend to talk. These gestures may seem relatively small to anyone who has never fought a battle with depression, but inside, they reflect a major thawing of the overwhelming numbness. According to Brown and Harris (1978) the reintroduction of normality is what signals recovery. For me, it was funny to feel excitement over a silly show on Netflix or a low-key brunch on the horizon: "Wow, I actually want to do something." Depression's lie that wanting was impossible started falling apart.

There were relapses, lasting days or even weeks, when the darkness returned in full force. Nonetheless, each relapse felt slightly more bearable since I had learnt coping skills, relied on supportive friends, and had a track record of successfully pulling myself out before. If a slump murmured, "You're back at square one," I might respond, "No, I was here three weeks ago and emerged. "I can do it again.".

Key Takeaways

- Depression doesn't always mean dramatic crying: Many days, it's a numb and energy-drained state that feels huge just to get basic tasks done (NIMH, 2018)

- Small Steps Matter: Even minor behavioral activation, a five-minute stroll or a short text can circumvent inertia (Jacobson et al., 2001). It can be hard to summon the energy, but little victories lead to bigger ones.

- Routine and Social Contact Help: Regular sleep schedules and light, social exercise provide stability to mood (Dimidjian et al., 2014). Socializing, even slightly, helps offset the amplifying effects of isolation on depression (Hammen, 2018).

- Soothing Humor: Gently ridiculing negative thoughts or using humorous frames can disrupt ruminative cycles (Beck & Emery, 1985). Self-compassion encourages resilience (Neff, 2011), that means treating yourself as kindly as you would a friend.

- Professional Help: These severe cases usually require therapy, medication, or both, and these can truly save lives. A safety plan can list contacts and simple grounding acts, like watch a silly cat video or call a trusted buddy.

- Healing Isn't Linear: Prepare for highs and lows. Temporary setbacks do not negate overall progress (Beck, 1976).

- A Gradual Glimmer of Hope: Slowly, small wins, such as getting to eat a favorite meal, signal depression's hold is loosening. This generates fresh empathy and perspective, which ironically makes you more understanding of the struggles of others (Jamison, 1995).

Emerging from depression is less a glorious sprint than an uphill slog. If anxiety can, at times, be soothed by immediate grounding, depression demands a softer, patiently relentless touch. All those little acts, taking a few steps, engaging in a bit of dialogue, are a defiant proclamation that you are not giving up. Because although the path is rarely just up and up, the joke is how little, almost wastefully, doing something (like doodling for 10 minutes) can diminish depression's grip. f you're in that quicksand, remember that even a dim sense of hope is still hope. As Dr. Nguyen often reminded me: "You are not stuck forever. Depression is lying." That lie can be exposed by persistent, incremental evidence that your life is worth engaging with.

Each small step or laugh or shared meal proves there's more to you than numbness. And as we go on, in the next Chapter 9, the art of "Failing Spectacularly", we shift our focus outward to how resilience and humor help us bounce back from outer setbacks, just as they help us rise from inner struggles. If we can find our footing against depression's weight, can't we also risk a few glorious flops in life's bigger arena, confident we can get up again? Let's find out.

Chapter 9: Failing Spectacularly

Failure is the blooper reel in life's highlight show. If you can
laugh at it, you're already halfway to success.

Failure. Just reading that word can tighten your chest a bit, can't it? From childhood onward, many of us learn to associate failure with shame, falling short of good grades, losing games, missing that promotion. Yet if you watch commencement speeches or scroll motivational quotes online, you'll often see lines like "Fail forward!" or "Failure is the best teacher!" It's a strange contradiction: culturally, we discourage failure, but philosophically, we treasure it as essential for growth. In this chapter, I want to reconcile that tension with a wink and a nudge, because, ironically, we might need to fail at the fear of failure to truly flourish.

The Hall of Famous Failures (and Myths)

Let us begin with the "famous failures" of motivational literature. While some of these details might be exaggerated, those stories are emblematic of a larger truth: Errors can often lay the groundwork for glorious achievement.

Legend has it that before he invented the filament for the electric light bulb, Thomas Edison tried many different materials. He is frequently quoted as saying, "I have not failed. "I just discovered 10,000 ways that didn't work." Baldwin (1995) does not make it clear how many times he was tested but best test results overall. The exact origins of the specific quotation are murky, and the number may be symbolic or exaggerated at that. To be sure, his lab notes reflect much trial and error, indicating that he viewed each "flop" as a sign of progress. That goofy mindset re-casts failures as data entries and not personal failures.

J. K. Rowling, the "Harry Potter" author, faced a slew of publisher rejections before finding a "Yes." Some accounts say she was turned away a dozen times; others provide slightly different numbers. J.K. Rowling's commencement speech, delivered in 2008 at Harvard, yet another example of personal experience and struggle being a strong fuel to persistence, despite all the pain caused (Rowling, 2008). The humor is that had she stopped at rejection 6 or 9, the Wizarding World phenomena probably wouldn't have happened.

Most of the time, we only enjoy "disasters" after they turn out to be successes, even though they can be very upsetting at the time. In fact, being turned down or criticized can hurt your self-esteem. But humor can help change how we think about loss, making it less painful and more open to new ideas. Laughing at your mistakes can help you learn from them instead of dwelling on your flaws, which will help you move forward more effectively in the long run.

Failure does not need to be final

Humans may not be as much inspired by their own failures as we think. A study by Eskreis-Winkler and Fishbach (2019) conducted at the University of Chicago found that self-examination of successes provides more instructional insight than self-examination of failures. This feedback is painful and not well received, so the ego tries to avoid failure at all costs which cripples growth and performance. The researchers explain that because our sense of ourselves will not be threatened when we see other people fail, we are open to learning important lessons.

What do we do to get past our ego? One way to do this is to embrace a growth mindset, (Dweck, 2006). If you see abilities as flexible, failures can guide you toward how to improve. A more creative tool is comedic distancing. Pretend your flop is a showreel of the funniest outtakes ever. By making a joke, it creates an emotional distance which gives a way to analyze it objectively without the emotions of shame.

Learning From Failure: Easier Said Than Done

If life were Scrubs, your flops would be the goofy outtakes at the season wrap party. These so-called "bloopers" are often met with laughter because they showcase real, human moments. The joke is, we all have little cringes in the stash, like accidentally calling your boss "Mom" or tripping close to the crush you're in love with, or a dinner party that has gone so badly that smoke alarms go off. These painful experiences, when the redness passes, make fantastic stories and can, if we are willing to scrutinize them, even spur future achievement.

The Fail-Fast Philosophy

The term fail-fast is somewhat of a mantra within IT and entrepreneurial circles (Ries, 2011). The concept is to fail very quickly, understand that with many inventions you'll fail, and pivot quickly to see what doesn't work. Failure is a chance to learn as opposed to a conclusive verdict. One example from history that will make you smile is when 3M invented the Post-it Note. A 3M scientist working on a super-strong glue accidentally created a low-tack type instead. A colleague thought it appropriate for bookmarks they don't write on pages. There's a Post-it note. In fact, 3M's famous Post-it product was a byproduct of this "bootlegging" mentality according to hook studies (Fry, 1986) and was initially considered to be a show of jest of failed products and side-initiation. Had the founding crew complained of the "failed glue," this unusual and sticky product may not have ended up on the market.

A Hypothetical Startup Adventure: BrightIdea Inc.

A fictional firm, BrightIdea Inc., whose leader is a starry-eyed entrepreneur convinced that her new program would change the world. Failure can lead to success. The first app is buggy, the second pivot flops with investors, and team morale plummets. Nina will "celebrate" every debacle with humor and turn guilt into a shared lesson.

Crash-o-Matic Application: The first product malfunctions after 30 seconds of use. Nina has a "Failure Party." The developer adds in jest that the software also serves as a phone hand warmer and "trains user patience with endless loading spinners." It also makes them identify flaws like too many features and leaks in memory and find solutions to fix it. Freed of shame, they heal in a less biased way.

The Investor Rejection Reel: The second pivot gets a no thanks from VC Nina goes the "Wall of Nope" route, a vitriolic mosaic of harsh hues. And that comic pitch turns antagonism into a roast that the team can appraise from a distance, calling out durable weaknesses in the process. They simplify their product concept after identifying user pain points.

Near Zero Cash: By Year 3, there wasn't enough potential for growth in the third variant. And in the wake of a big transition, a major project has a six-month time frame. "Even if we screw up again," Nina tells the crew with a chuckle, "at least we'll have hilarious stories to share at our reunion down the road." She plays a slideshow of "Epic Fails of BrightIdea," including the initial crash and embarrassing comments from investors. The funny oracle reminds them that they've survived other calamities, and that this, too, sunless moment is not the end of the world.

Let us say BrightIdea Inc. gets some new money and has some small success. They make failing funny, which is good for learning, improves skills, and creates a safe space for people to fail, even if they don't. Edmondson (1999) says that a culture of openness and "smart honesty" pushes people to work together, talk about their mistakes, and come up with new ideas. By making weekly fails into fun "roasts," the team stays flexible and doesn't mind learning from their mistakes.

Failures, Big and Small

Not all failures are as monumental as a full startup crash, and many are felt on a personal level that is limited to us or our close friends. Failing an exam or burning a romantic dinner or botching a job interview may not make headlines, but the sting is real. Here, humor and perspective still matter.

A failed interview, for example, could become an anecdote: "I was so nervous that I literally invented a new language halfway through the interview because my nerves jumble my thoughts." Over coffee with a friend, you can poke fun at yourself while getting insights into what you did wrong (lack of prep, maybe, or a mismatch with the company's culture). No longer shackled to the ego's whine, "I'm worthless," you can pivot to "I can do better in the next."

The pain of relationship failures is more emotional. A breakup or a night that ends awkwardly can hurt for weeks. Mirth should never cheapen heartbreak, but there are times it can help you shuffle around the jagged pain. When you are ready, turning framing that disastrous date as a comedic story, like "he spent half the date showing me cat memes in silence!", makes you see it less as a personal failing and more as a weird occurrence. According to relationship researcher Gottman (Gottman & Silver, 2012), couples who approach conflict with levity are more durable. And those able to chuckle softly on love-life fails may adjust faster.

Embracing the "FAIL" Label

The internet culture has partially stripped the word fail of its venom, applying it to ordinary follies: "Epic fail!" or "FAIL" for comedic effect. We can take that approach in our personal lives. React to cringe-worthy behavior, literally calling it "Well, that was a fail!" can anticipate your inner critic. Calling out the mistake verbally helps you take ownership of the error rather than allowing the error to define you. And this comedic acceptance can help quell shame, so you can look at the fiasco more dispassionately. To extract the most lessons from a mistake, we need to confront the feedback head-on (Eskreis-Winkler & Fishbach, 2019). If we cover it with shame, we echo it. Normalizing the word "fail" removes some of the emotional charge, making it easier to disassemble. If that mental reel rewinds to replay, "I messed up," it is far less toxic if you append a comedic wink: "I messed up spectacularly, let's see how I can come back and do better next time."

The Science of Bouncing Back

A growing body of evidence shows that repeated failure can lead to eventual success, but only if each failure leads to adaptation. (Wang et al., 2013) argue that people (or teams) who keep iterating after each failure often eventually cross a "tipping point", after which the iteration crosses a threshold leading to success. The funny or reassuring bit is that the distance between repeated fails and instantaneous success can be a straight line: a pressure cooker that eventually finds its sweet spot.

Still, the comedic disclaimers hold, not all failures lead to breakthroughs, and not everyone who fails will eventually succeed. Repeated failure, at times, means changing track or resetting ambitions. According to Edmonson (1999), "the question of why any given failure occurred, for instance, due to a bad strategy, lack of a capacity, or environmental pressures, informs whether you continue iterating or pivot." Humor protects you from that analysis by softening the blow.

Looping through Infinite Schemes: From Failing to

Flailing

"Fail forward" doesn't mean stupendously making the same mistakes. If your same screw-up million-times a day is the same, it's not a funny story, it's bad. In fact, a sense of humor about failures is most effective paired with sincere reflection. "I messed up, haha, let's see if I can do better," not "I messed up, haha, oh well, I'm going to do the same thing tomorrow."

The theory points out that perseverance added with the analysis leads to improvement (Duckworth, 2016). If you keep failing in the same way, you may be ignoring the feedback. If you try a different method each time and fail in a new way, in a way that implies an experimental effort, you might be on a path forward. The comic twist being that a new class of errors can show you're evolving your strategy rather than mired in the status quo.

A Personal Montage: Navigating Embarrassment

Think of your own catalog of flops: a tray dropped in a cafeteria, an insulting comment to a friend when you meant to simply bulk-up joke, a failing grade in a class you'd hoped you could get A's in. The comic or cinematic version would be a montage to an upbeat song, your younger self tripping here, your senior self-mishandling there, pausing on each frame. Slowly link one cringe moment to the major shift in your behavior or your awareness that was to arrive.

The humor part is that in the end, the irony is that that chaos often makes for the most relatable, lovable part of your story. Which is the sort of thing that family reunions or friend reunions frequently center on reciting these comedic fail stories like that time you tried to clear a sink and flooded the kitchen instead. If you can also generalize their results, you'll be able to learn from them.' You can build up the resolve to pursue loftier goals if you grow from them.

How to Own Your Failures and Reap the Rewards

Failing is scary when we view it as the ultimate judgment on our competence. But if we think about failure as a pratfall on life's stage with possibilities for punch line, we turn shame into curiosity. We can take a step back and ask, "What did I do wrong and how can I adjust?" instead of allowing the fiasco engulf us."

In chapter 10, we'll examine the next dimension: relationships, and how we change as we connect with others. We'll discover that such comic acceptance of missteps can also repair or fortify social relationships, because everybody trips up sometimes. Until then, remember that flops can not only teach valuable lessons, but may well make up your best party stories down the line. If you can make a joke about your misfire, you're on your way to peeking into its wisdom.

Key Takeaways

- Failure Is Universal but Stigmatized: We are raised fearing failure, we will top our classes and get the promotion, but the stories of success contain devastating failures (the 10,000 tests of Edison, the rejections of Rowling). The tension is comedic because we are told to fear failure, but also to learn from it.

- Famous Failures Inspire: Before a groundbreaking single tear moment, comes a series of spine crunching rejections (Baldwin, 1995; Rowling, 2008). They remind us that one (or a dozen) "No's" don't determine our final destination.

- Learning From Our Own Fails Isn't Automatic: People tend to not learn from their own mistakes because it stings their egos (Eskreis-Winkler & Fishbach, 2019). Ironically, we learn more from others' failures than from our own.

- Repeating the Same Mistakes = Tragedy, Not Comedy: "Fail forward" doesn't mean ignoring feedback. True iteration requires analyzing each flop's cause (Edmonson, 1999) and trying different fixes (Duckworth, 2016)

- Fail Fast but Reflect: It is through instilling failure that they create breakthroughs (Ries, 2011). The Post-it Note story and (Wang et al., 2013) theory of "tipping points" perfectly illustrates how so many flops can drive us straight to the goldmine, as long as we iterate with humor.

- Failures Vary in Scale: Not every flop is a spectacular corporate failure. Sometimes you just fall in front of your crush. You are not party to data at work, but humor still apply in misadventures personal, jest invites endurance.

- Own the "FAIL" Label: Internet slang transmutes fails to comic bites: "Epic fail!" Carrying that attitude through life then is a good way to bypass your inner critic. By owning your slip up with a chuckle, you take back agency over it.

- Analyze, Don't Repeat Blindly: "Fail forward" is not an objection to learning from your mistakes. You must refine. Otherwise, it's just a circle of farcical destruction. And, Perseverance (Duckworth, 2016) + comedic reflection equals genuine improvement.

Failing can be terrifying if we view it as a final verdict on our competence. But if we reinterpret failure as a comedic slip-on life's stage, complete with a clown cameo or a meltdown cameo, we transform shame into curiosity. Suddenly, a fiasco isn't "I'm worthless" but "That was silly, how do I do better?"

In Chapter 10, we'll shift from these personal or professional fiascos to see how relationships factor into deeper transformations. Humor and acceptance of missteps can mend or strengthen bonds because, after all, everyone fails sometimes. For now, remember: a fiasco can become your funniest party story, as well as your biggest teacher, if you embrace it with a comedic wink and a growth-oriented gaze.

Chapter 10: Relationships and the Art of Humor

Relationships are like comedic duets. Sometimes you nail the harmony, sometimes you step on each other's toes, but the shared laughter keeps the act on stage

Relationships, whether romantic partnerships, friendships, or family ties, often loom in our minds as "serious business." We're told they require communication, compromise, or "hard work," which is all true, but seldom do people put "laughter" at the top of the requirement list. Yet if you think about your dearest connections, there's a good chance laughter frequently weaves through them. Something about a shared joke or an unexpected pun creates closeness that few other things can match (Kurtz & Algoe, 2015).

Robert Waldinger, director of the Harvard Study of Adult Development, famously reported that strong, healthy relationships are some of the best predictors of long-term happiness and even physical health (Waldinger, 2016). This study, which began in 1938 and spanned over eight decades, repeatedly found that the quality of our social bonds matters more than wealth or fame for living a fulfilling life. If bonds protect us from stress and help us thrive, then humor is often their unsung hero, like a comedic backstage crew ensuring the show runs smoothly (Butzer & Kuiper, 2008).

But another curious fact remains. How a lighthearted approach, an apt joke, or the ability to find hilarity in everyday routines can strengthen relationships? And the next paragraphs, go beyond arguing that Love may make the world go 'round, but as these pages argue, humor keeps us from getting dizzy.

The Couple That Laughs Together, Lasts Together

An older couple who's been together for decades, they might bicker, but often they have developed a shorthand of jokes, gentle ribbing, and mutual silliness. The Association for Psychological Science suggests couples who incorporate humor report higher relationship satisfaction (APS, 2024). The comedic side is that with one knowing smirk or pun, they can communicate an entire subtext: the memory of that time the smoke alarm went off at midnight or the inside joke about Dad's mispronunciation of a newfangled gadget.

Shared Laughter as "We-ness"

Laughter fosters a sense of closeness and "we-ness." Psychologists label this "overlapping sense of self," suggesting that when you and another person find the same thing funny, it signals a mini "aha!" moment: we see the world similarly(Kurtz & Algoe, 2015). Humor demands a certain empathy, knowing what tickles your partner or friend. Couples who develop a playful banter or silly nicknames demonstrate that they understand each other in an affectionate, often idiosyncratic, way.

The Stress Buffer Effect

Couples inevitably face challenges, financial worries, health issues, or childcare demands. Humor offers relief (Ziv, 2010). In a comedic scenario, two underslept new parents could become foes at 3:00 a.m. or could share a delirious laugh about raising a tiny overlord. That moment of mirth reaffirms being on the same team as a couple, a bond that can serve as emotional armor against life's stressors.

It's been said that humor is "five times more important than physical intimacy" for a happy marriage, but there is no study that backs up that claim. But the main point is clear: humor is always high on lists of qualities that people want in a partner (Butzer & Kuiper, 2008). We don't have to stick to an unproven number; instead, we can rely on well-researched facts and personal experience. In fact, many couples find that having the same sense of humor is more important than other, more surface-level things when it comes to keeping their relationship healthy and long-lasting.

Why Humor Eases Relationship Friction

Relational friction arises over minor annoyances, someone constantly leaving the toilet seat up, or being late, or chewing too loudly. These repeated irritations can fester into big conflicts or become comedic fodder. The difference often lies in the approach. If you can adopt a playful tone, "Good morning, my dear Shoeless Wonder; I see you left your sneakers in the hallway again!", the frustration can be delivered without venom. Research on positive communication in marriages suggests that humor can diffuse defensiveness, leading to more constructive outcomes (Gottman & Silver, 2012).

The comedic side is that a small shift in tone, gentle grin vs. pointed sarcasm, can determine if the message lands safely or ignites a quarrel. Obviously, meanness disguised as "joking" can be toxic. The aim is gentle humor that invites the other person to laugh, not to feel belittled.

Case Study: Dollars and Sense (of Humor)

Finances often rank among couples' top stressors. Let's meet Priya (the saver) and David (the spender). Typically, each big unplanned expense leads to arguments, bruised egos, and tension. But one day, upon discovering David's pricey new golf clubs, Priya tries humor: she dresses up as a fake "Budget Caddy" with brooms over her shoulder, announcing, "Hello, Mr. Golfer! Might I recommend a deposit into our rainy-day fund to complement these shiny clubs?"

The Budget Caddy Skit

One day, Priya notices a credit card charge labeled "Dave's Deluxe Golf Emporium." David has dropped a large sum on new golf clubs. Instead of confronting him angrily, Priya decides to try humor. That evening, she saunters into the living room dressed as a "Budget Caddy," brooms slung over her shoulder like clubs. In a cheerful, mock-professional voice, she says, "Why, hello, Mr. Golfer! Might I suggest balancing this new driver with a nice deposit into our vacation fund?"

David bursts out laughing, instantly disarmed. By turning an impending argument into playful theatrics, Priya has short-circuited David's usual defensiveness. Freed from tension, they talk real numbers. She gently expresses, "I'd appreciate a heads-up on big purchases," while also acknowledging his desire for fun money. David sheepishly admits he got carried away, but jokes that a caddy is essential for his "tour champion lifestyle." They settle on an arrangement: David will consult Priya for major expenses, while Priya will let David have a small "discretionary spending" pot each month.

"Should we call the Budget Caddy on that Amazon cart?" they might joke after a while. It turns out that inside joke is a friendly way to bring up something that used to be controversial. Studies on dyadic coping (Bodenmann et al., 2006) show that using positive and funny tactics during fights can make the relationship better. This shows how to handle a big issue, like spending too much, without getting into a fight.

Friends and Family: Humor Binds Groups

Romantic couples aren't the only beneficiaries. Humor can significantly deepen friendships and family ties. Many of our strongest memories with close friends revolve around cracking each other up over something silly. That shared laughter forges a sense of belonging (Butzer & Kuiper, 2008). Inside jokes become membership tokens in the tribe.

In families, humor can bridge age or cultural gaps. A grandparent might not understand a teenager's slang, but one well-timed comedic remark can connect them in seconds. Siblings, too, often preserve a small library of teasing nicknames and comedic references from childhood. Even workplaces can harness the comedic vibe. A dash of humor among colleagues fosters camaraderie, so long as it's done respectfully (Holmes & Marra, 2002). A manager who occasionally deploys self-deprecating humor can appear more approachable, promoting an environment of psychological safety.

The Healing Side of Laughter

Some therapists help families devise "healing humor," using comic relief to signal a reset after conflict, the way you see so many family groups in sitcoms break humor. For example, a few counselors recommend scheduling something goofy, like a "family costume night" or goofy charades, to remind everyone that they can have fun together, even if they just argued over chores or finances. Laughter is often an indication of forgiveness or at least a willingness to move on. This comedic chemistry cultivates the idea, "We'd rather be happy together than mad at each other."

When Humor Backfires

All of this, of course, comes with a caveat: Humor in relationships is dangerous. It is not a cure all, and timing is important (Gottman & Silver, 2012). If someone is very upset, hurling jokes right away may feel dismissive: "Oh, you're not taking me seriously?" Humor works best pending a nod to seriousness or an opening.

Again, everyone has different comedic styles. If they hit you in a sensitive spot, or sound belittling, sarcastic jokes can cut. A "silly" comment about someone's weight or intelligence might shatter trust instead of strengthening it. It's generally a wise rule of comedic thumb that it is better to laugh at yourself or the situation than the other person. Self-deprecating humor can be disarming, but there's a fine line to tread, because if it becomes the routine, and you keep poking fun of your partner's quirks, it can become negative.

If, for instance, instead, Priya had mocked David with, period "Wow, Mr. Moneybags, is your ego that huge?" perhaps in a mocking tone, one that'd likely elicit defensiveness instead of constructive conversation. But that variance in tone could make the difference between a comedic invitation and a personal attack.

The path to bonding: a shared journey

At its core, if humor in relationships is built on anything, it's the idea: we're in this together. If you can laugh with someone you remind yourselves that you both have a vantage point, however temporary. It's not "me vs. you"; it's "us vs. the problem" or "us vs. life's chaos." That unity is potent. Actually, an 80-year Harvard Study of adult development found that it was the warmth of relationships, cradled by shared positive emotions, that was the top predictor of happiness and longevity (Waldinger, 2016). Laughter in particular can be the glue that spans the rough patches that relationships inevitably experience.

The life that throws us curvies can seem less menacing when we are laughing uproariously together. A financial meltdown, a health scare, an exhausting job, these are serious. But relationships that include some humor usually navigate them better. If you can laugh together about the unpredictable nature of existence, you're more likely to have each other's back.

So how can you add more humor to your relationships?

- Make Your Own Inside Jokes: It may be a goofy reference to the time you both locked yourselves out of the house or a funny name for a mutual pet peeve. Such jokes are emotional shorthand, like comic glue, for deeper intimacy.
- Celebrate Quirks: If your partner incessantly loses their keys, you might jokingly line them up on a "lost-and-found" shelf and post a sign. When done softly, it's a nudge not a nag.
- Use "We-Against-It" Language: The next time life serves up a pile of stress, try to spin a comic "It's us against this crazy day!" approach. By personifying adversity as the comedic villain, you and your friend or partner become one.
- Be Kind: Keep jokes no barbed. Don't take yourself (or life) so seriously. If a loved one says "That's not funny," take them at their word.
- Make Some Fun Happen: Watch a comedy special or do some silly activity. A good joke or ten minutes of laughter together can lighten things. There's a reason "laughter yoga" groups exist (even if that's a pun, rather than the literal kind of stretch).

And yes, sure, these might taste a little contrived in the beginning, but relationships often thrive on that nudge of deliberate positive feeling (Fredrickson, 2001). One positivity hack is humor.

Case Study: The Sisterly Prank Original

Another example using a fictitious set of sisters: two sickly sweet sisters, Jana and Melissa, in their mid-twenties. They bicker often about chores. Jana says she's a neat-freak, and Melissa leaves piles of laundry. More free-spirited Melissa resents Jana's tireless "tidy tyranny." Usually, their arguments end in sulking or door-slamming.

Original Case Study: The Sisterly Prank

Another hypothetical scenario: two sisters, Jana and Melissa, living together in their mid-twenties. They frequently clash over chores. Jana, a neat freak, complains that Melissa leaves laundry piles. Melissa, more free-spirited, resents Jana's endless "tidy tyranny." Typically, their arguments escalate into sulking or door-slamming.

The "Laundry Monster" Stunt

One weekend, Jana decides on comedic remedy. She compiles Melissa's scattered laundry into a mock "monster" in Melissa's room, a heap topped with a silly face drawn on cardboard. Jana leaves a note: "Greetings from the Laundry Monster! I'm hungry for a hamper, rawr!" Melissa stumbles upon it, bursts out laughing, and calls Jana, "You absolute weirdo." Jana retorts, "Just feed your monster, please."

They talk it out while giggling. Jana gently explains that while tidiness is vital for her mental clarity, she won't pester Melissa if Melissa commits to a hamper system. Melissa concedes, "Okay, I'll hamper it up, just no more midnight monster raids!" The comedic approach diffuses the usual tension. Soon, "the Laundry Monster's hungry again!" becomes an inside joke.

Results? Jana feels less frustration, Melissa feels less nagged. The comedic approach fosters empathy: Jana conveys the annoyance in a playful, not accusatory, manner. Melissa sees the fun side of the chore complaints. Possibly they still argue sometimes, but the comedic lens offers a friendlier route to resolution.

When Humor Runs Thin

Of course, not all issues can be resolved by comedic stunts alone. Some conflicts, like deep betrayals or systemic problems, demand serious discussion, possibly therapy. Humor can't fix profound trauma or major compatibility problems. Used skillfully, it's a supplement to real communication, not a replacement. If Jana and Melissa had more severe issues, like financial entanglements or lifestyle conflicts, they might need direct conversation or professional mediation.

Also, individuals differ in comedic taste. Some appreciate goofy antics, others favor witty banter, and some are easily offended by sarcasm or teasing (Butzer & Kuiper, 2008). The comedic approach thrives best in a relationship where both parties share or respect each other's humor boundaries.

Key Takeaways

- Humor Reinforces Bonds: Sharing a lighthearted moment fosters a sense of unity. Kurtz & Algoe (2015) suggests that couples who laugh together build a deeper "we-ness." It's not trivial, laughter can be the invisible thread tying two people closer.

- Playfulness Beats Tension: From new parents coping with exhaustion to siblings bickering over chores, comedic reframing can turn irritations into comedic fodder, easing conflict (Gottman & Silver, 2012). Proper tone and empathy ensure it remains uplifting, not hurtful.

- It's Not Just About Couples: Friendships and families thrive on humor too, shared jokes create a sense of "in-group" identity. Workplace teams can improve morale through lighthearted banter, as long as it stays inclusive (Holmes & Marra, 2002).

- Serious Doesn't Cancel Funny: Handling heavy issues (health crises, financial woes) can be aided by a well-timed laugh that reminds you you're in it together. The comedic approach doesn't trivialize serious topics; it supplies a momentary relief that can spark cooperation (Ziv, 2010).

- Know the Boundaries: Sarcasm or teasing about sensitive topics can harm trust. The comedic approach must be gentle, affectionate, or self-deprecating. Hitting a raw nerve with "It's just a joke!" can worsen negativity (Gottman & Silver, 2012).

- The Best Medicine? While the old adage "laughter is the best medicine" can be hyperbole, some problems need more direct solutions, humor certainly helps keep spirits afloat. Combining comedic positivity with direct communication is often a potent formula for relationship satisfaction (Fredrickson, 2001).

- Tethered to Longevity: The famous Harvard Adult Development study found that the warmth of relationships is key to happiness and health (Waldinger, 2015). Humor helps cultivate that warmth, potentially extending both emotional and physical well-being.

- A Light-Hearted Invitation: No need to wait for the fight to start. Sprinkle your daily interactions with gentle humor, pet names, comedic references to inside jokes, so that when the friction does arise, you've got a well of good will and comedic "secret code" stored to come back to.

Romantic, familial or platonic, relationships gain unexpected strength from humor. It's an underappreciated superpower that creates intimacy, diffuses conflicts and reconfigures heavy loads into light chunks. From comedic rants about stray sneakers to jovial roastings over golf-club buys, the laughter is the hallmark of "We're in this together."

In the next Chapter 11, another dimension of interpersonal growth pops up: how ignorance, fear, and illusions can sometimes undermine our best intentions, and what mindful strategies might enable us to gain more clarity. If Chapter 10's humor taught us how to lighten up with our loved ones, Chapter 11 invites us to realize how our illusions of ourselves or another block true connection.

Chapter 11: Better Safe Than Sorry

It's good to have a helmet in life, but if you're wearing three helmets, five kneepads, and bubble wrap just to step outside, maybe 'safe' has gone too far.

From childhood on, most of us hear the proverb "Better safe than sorry," conjuring mental images of seatbelts, double-locking doors, or re-checking the stove before bed. And let's be honest, none of these actions are inherently bad. In many contexts, caution is wise. Indeed, we have modern aviation regulations, thorough pharmaceutical trials, and the ubiquitous seatbelt mandate partly because people once said, "We wish we'd been more careful."

Yet the paradox emerges when we consider the cost of too much caution. Humans flourish by taking reasonable leaps, whether launching new businesses or forging new friendships. Overdo the safety factor, and you might stay in your cocoon so thoroughly that you miss out on experiences. In this chapter, we'll analyze the tension between "be prudent" and "dare a little," exploring how the vantage might help us know when we're safer than necessary, and possibly sorrier for it.

The Case for Caution

Let's begin by giving caution its due. Much of modern society's progress rests on learning from past tragedies and implementing measures to avoid them. Airplanes have redundant systems to prevent catastrophic failure (International Civil Aviation Organization [ICAO], 2019). Pharmaceutical drugs go through extensive phases of testing because we'd rather be safe than sorry about side effects (U.S. Food and Drug Administration [FDA], 2024). Entrepreneurs who research their market and plan for the worst often fare better than those who gamble on gut feeling alone (Ries, 2011).

In daily life, caution can literally save your life: wearing a biking helmet is a trivial cost but may prevent severe brain injury (Thompson, Rivara, & Thompson, 2018). "Better safe than sorry" reflects the idea that a small precaution can avert a large regret. We teach kids to look both ways before crossing the street because the cost of a moment's vigilance is small compared to the risk of a car accident.

When "Safe" Is Actually Smart

Consider the scenario of texting while driving. The upside? Sending a quick message. The downside? A possible crash. Clearly, the stakes are too high. Taking the vantage, you might say, "Better to be 10 seconds late to respond than 10 weeks in a cast." People who ignore these cautionary principles often supply the "fail" videos we see, but the outcome can be tragic. So in high-stakes contexts, like driving, nuclear power, or extreme sports, "better safe than sorry" stands firmly as wise policy (Russell & Blowers, 2013).

Overcaution: When Safety Becomes a Vice

Yet caution can morph into paralysis if we let fear become the deciding factor. Kodak's infamous story is a classic corporate cautionary tale: despite inventing a prototype digital camera in 1975, Kodak hesitated to pivot away from film, fearing it would cannibalize their core business (Lucas & Goh, 2009). That caution ironically led them to miss the digital revolution. The irony? By "playing it safe," they sealed their downfall, a different kind of "sorry."

The vantage is that sometimes the "safe route" is the truly risky route. By avoiding new technology or business models, organizations can become obsolete. The moral is: "better safe than sorry" is wise for preventing catastrophic harm, but harmful if it means ignoring necessary innovation. Or as a more saying goes: The biggest risk is never taking any risk.

Everyday Caution: Good or Bad?

Now, let's pan to daily life. "Better safe than sorry" usually means not taking a chance that could lead to serious regret, like driving under the influence or ignoring a hurricane evacuation order. However, in lower-stakes arenas, over-caution can yield a subtler regret: missed opportunities. For instance, not applying to your dream job because you fear rejection or not asking out someone you genuinely like because you fear embarrassment. These "safe" routes might save you a bit of pain today, but in the long run you might feel sorrier about the chance you never took (Gilovich & Medvec, 1995).

Researchers Gilovich and Medvec (1995) note that short-term regrets revolve around actions that failed, but over a lifetime, people more often lament the risks they didn't take. The angle is that many seniors, asked about life regrets, say something like, "I wish I'd gone for it." So "better safe than sorry" can ironically lead to a deeper sorry if we systematically avoid growth or potential joy.

Overprotection: "Safe" but Sorry Later

Parenting is a domain where "better safe than sorry" is extremely common. Parents, driven by love, often shield kids from all conceivable risks: no playing in the street, no talking to strangers, sometimes no going outside unsupervised at all (Gray, 2013). But child-development experts warn that helicopter parenting, excessive protective oversight, can undermine resilience. If a child never experiences moderate risk or small failures, they may fail to learn coping strategies.

Psychologist Peter Gray (2013) notes that children need unstructured play to test boundaries, scraping a knee occasionally but discovering independence in the process.

Bubble-wrapped childhood has either a humorous or sad result: a young adult who lacks the ability to negotiate danger or disappointment panics at little difficulty. Ungar (2012) hypothesizes that overprotected children are more prone to experience anxiety or dependency problems. Although no one is arguing that young children should balance knives "for character-building," a calibrated approach permitting age-appropriate freedoms can help to promote competence. If it keeps youngsters from developing practical skills, "better safe than sorry" can cause more grief.

Corporate and Creative Worlds

The same "safe vs. sorry" dynamic manifests in innovation. Companies that cling to the status quo may avoid short-term failure but risk long-term irrelevance (Ries, 2011). Conversely, reckless risk can bankrupt a startup overnight. The vantage is seeing bright entrepreneurs pivot so fast they forget to do basic market research or "due diligence," leading to crash-and-burn stories. Real success demands calculated leaps: "Plan for the worst, hope for the best" (Russell & Blowers, 2013).

When "Safe" Bites You Back

In certain scenarios, extreme caution ironically causes exactly what we aimed to avoid. Suppose someone so terrified of heartbreak refuses to commit to any relationship, eventually ending up lonely, which is heartbreak of another kind. Or a germaphobe who sanitizes everything might weaken their immune system, making them more prone to illnesses (Bloomfield et al., 2006).

By never letting ourselves face mild adversity, we remain fragile. Like muscle training, our emotional or immune systems need a small dose of stress to become robust. Avoiding all challenges can produce a scenario of "over-safety," but with the sad result of missed personal growth or eventual meltdown at the slightest risk (Gray, 2013).

The Social Dimension of Overcaution

Sometimes "better safe than sorry" is used as an excuse for prejudicial avoidance, like skipping an entire neighborhood or profiling certain individuals. This might "feel safe," but the downside is it perpetuates ignorance, fear, or discrimination. If you never interact with anyone outside your comfort zone, your worldview shrinks, ironically making you less adaptable (Russell & Blowers, 2013). True safety is achieved through knowledge-based caution, not blanket avoidance.

The Middle Path

So how do we honor the spirit of "better safe than sorry" while avoiding stagnation or paranoia? A few points:

- Assess Likelihood and Severity: If both the likelihood and severity of a bad outcome are high. Like a potential car crash, lean heavily on caution (Thompson et al., 2018). If the likelihood is low or consequences mild, weigh the cost of caution carefully. Many of us overestimate rare dangers (Tversky & Kahneman, 1974).

- Consider Opportunity Cost: Playing it safe often carries a hidden price. Like missing a once-in-a-lifetime trip or not starting that dream business. Evaluate whether the risk is moderate enough to justify the potential reward (Gilovich & Medvec, 1995).

- Use Safety Nets: Want to start a business but fear losing your livelihood? Keep your day job initially, small tests reduce worst-case scenarios (Ries, 2011). This honors "better safe" while still striving for gains.

- Leverage Lessons: The proverb partly says, "Don't be sorry like others who weren't safe." Indeed, historical cautionary tales. Like seatbelts, nuclear meltdown precautions, underscore that ignoring clear risks can be deadly. Knowledge, not fear alone, should guide us.

- Moderation Is Gold: The twist is acknowledging that sometimes daring is better than dull. People differ in risk appetite, but a little spontaneity often spices life. Philosopher Bertrand Russell said, "To conquer fear is the beginning of wisdom." Over-sheltering can shrink your world.

Hypothetical Hurricane Mayors

Imagine a coastline town hearing that a hurricane might arrive in a week. One mayor says, "Better safe than sorry, evacuate everyone now!" If the hurricane veers away, this drastic measure wastes resources. Another mayor says, "It probably won't hit us," risking potential catastrophe. A balanced mayor might prepare shelters, track the forecast, and only evacuate with strong evidence. Balancing caution and proportionate response. A city bracing too soon, while everything remains calm; or ignoring warnings until the last second. The best approach splits the difference.

Key Takeaways

- Caution Has Its Place: "better safe than sorry" is wise for high-stakes, irreversible risks, like seatbelts, not diving headfirst into unfamiliar waters, or nuclear power checks (ICAO, 2019; FDA, 2024). A trivial precaution can avert disaster.

- Overprotection Yields Different Sorrows: Helicopter parenting can stunt kids' resilience (Gray, 2013). Corporate fear can lead to missed innovation (Kodak's example). Personal over-caution can block meaningful experiences. Sometimes the biggest risk is never taking any risk.

- Short-Term vs. Long-Term Regret: People often regret failed actions briefly, but over a lifetime, they regret missed chances more (Gilovich & Medvec, 1995). So "playing it safe" might prevent immediate "sorry," but cause deeper sorrow of inaction.

- Moderate Risk Grows Strength: Systems (like immune or emotional) often require mild stress to build resilience. Avoiding all risk can leave one fragile (Bloomfield et al., 2006). A vantage: bubble-wrapping yourself to avoid every scratch can ironically make you more vulnerable.

- Calculated Risk, Not Recklessness: Corporate or creative success merges caution (due diligence) with bold leaps (Ries, 2011). Same for personal endeavors: plan for downsides, have safety nets, but still go for it. Balance caution with adventure.

- Social Costs: Sometimes "better safe than sorry" justifies prejudice or ignorance, e.g., avoiding entire groups or neighborhoods (Russell & Blowers, 2013). True safety harnesses knowledge and rational risk assessment, not blanket fear.

- The Middle Path: Evaluate odds and severity of consequences, weigh opportunity costs, use backups, and learn from real cautionary tales. The difference between wise caution and paralyzing fear is recognizing when the risk is moderate enough to seize the moment.

So, "better safe than sorry" remains a valid principle in contexts where potential harm is grave or irreversible. Yet applying it indiscriminately can choke off spontaneity, growth, and resilience. If caution in Chapter 11 told us to protect ourselves from harm, Chapter 12 "Birds of a Feather Flock Together" will explore how our social or familial instincts pull us toward certain groups. How we gravitate to similar others for safety and identity. And what that means for diversity, innovation, and empathy.

Chapter 12: The Beauty of Doing Nothing

You might just discover hidden magic when you stop frantically trying to avoid doing nothing

Remember the last time you experienced genuine, undiluted boredom? Not the vexation of a page that took three seconds to load, but a deeper calm set by the absence of anything to do, no pressing to-do list, nothing with which to distract yourself. If you're like most people today, such moments are few and far between. Every moment of inaction can be filled with a swipe of a smartphone, a scroll, a tap. While having such entertainment at the ready is convenient, who doesn't love cat videos on demand?, we seldom permit ourselves to sink into real boredom. But boredom, as strange as that sounds, has untapped advantages: It can free up creativity, rest your mind and spark unexpected insights.

In this modern age, when apps and streaming services compete endlessly for our gaze, real boredom is dying out. Life is full of duties, notifications and recommendations, giving us little opportunity to sit around twiddling our thumbs. But in trading away that idle space, we may also be trading away an important mental commodity: the space to roam. This chapter offers a breezy, wry examination of why we flee from boredom and how "doing nothing" might actually be more precious than we realize. You may even recognize yourself in a scene or two, striking a stiff upper lip when all you want to do is check your phone or fill the vacuum with a "quick show." We'll learn that in an overstimulated world, deliberately engaging with boredom from time to time can lead to creativity, reflection and calm.

The "Never-Bored" Generation: Always On, Always

Distracted

Digital platforms compete to capture and use our time, grab our attention in what has come to be called the "Attention Economy" (Wu, 2016). Never-ending content scrolls, newscast feeds, and extremely engaging app designs all promote near-constant use. Standing in line at the supermarket? Whip out a phone. It's the middle of a show and it goes to commercial break? Grab the tablet. Pausing at a red light? Resist the rabbit hole of checking that message (please). If this sound slightly ridiculous, just think lots of people watching a streaming series on a TV device simultaneously browse social media on a phone, maybe also switching between a second screen with a message. Far from bored, we are often overstimulated.

Are we happier for it? Research indicates the connection is not that straightforward. Spending too much time on media can be associated with increased anxiety and reduced attention (Cheever, Rosen, Carrier, & Chavez, 2014). And ironically, the never-ending deluge of "stuff to do" creates a feeling of mental clutter. One reason we flinch so violently at boredom is that we've grown unaccustomed to allowing the mind to idle. In a striking 2014 experiment, researchers invited participants to sit by themselves with their thoughts for up to 15 minutes, no phone, no reading material. Many opted to give themselves mild electric shocks instead of sitting there alone in silence (Wilson et al., 2014). Being still was more distressing than a shot of little bit of pain.

That shocking outcome (quite literally) underscores how uneasy we have become with mental emptiness. The moment external stimulation fades, many of us scramble to fill the void. Yet in discarding boredom, we may also lose something subtle but powerful: the chance for new ideas and insights to bubble up.

Boredom and Creativity

Boredom can act like a signal for the brain, a subtle itch that says, "You're under-stimulated. Find or create something that engages you more meaningfully." People who never let themselves "space out" might perpetually snack on mental junk food, like endless social media scrolls, without addressing deeper creative or intellectual hungers. Several psychologists have argued that idle moments provide the backdrop for the "aha!" flash we associate with creative breakthroughs (Elpidorou, 2014). If your mind is too busy processing memes or clickbait, those flashes might remain buried.

A great example is the concept of "shower thoughts." You don't need full mental capacity to wash your hair, and so your mind is free to wander. Many have revelations under the shower head, everything from fresh scientific concepts to plot breakthroughs for a novel. Some great advances in art or science came about while daydreaming during a lull, historically. Archimedes' "Eureka!" attack may not have happened while he was racing around, but when he soaked and allowed his mind to wander. If we never unplug, we never drift into the mental space where surprising connections are made, in a modern sense. Allowing yourself to be bored, really bored, can free you from the treadmill of input, allowing original thoughts to rise up from the silence.

Boredom as a Signal, Not a Sin

Another aspect of boredom is that it can be a nudge to seek more purposeful action. If you always bury that nudge under quick digital hits, you risk missing a deeper call. A bored mind might prompt you to dust off an old guitar, plan a spontaneous meet-up with a friend you haven't seen in ages, or jot down early ideas for a novel you'd once dreamed of writing. In short, a mild sense of emptiness sometimes points to the desire for more meaningful engagement.

Without the chance to feel that itch, we might keep nibbling mental "snacks" (like endless cat videos) rather than sitting down to a meaningful "meal" (like learning an instrument or working on a passion project). Boredom, ironically, can be the impetus that propels us to move from mindless to mindful pursuits (Elpidorou, 2014).

The Cabin Experiment: A Tale of Idle Days

To illustrate the value of boredom, consider Alex and Bella, two college friends who tried a "boredom experiment" one spring break. They decided to unplug and retreat to a rustic cabin for three days: no internet, no TV, minimal entertainment. Just nature, basic art supplies, and a stack of old books. Bella, who was known for multi-screen consumption, quietly stashed her phone with downloaded shows "in case she cracked."

Day 1: Stir-Crazy Beginnings

Initially, the trip felt quaint. They slept in, cooked a leisurely breakfast. By midday, however, Bella began pacing around restlessly, opening the fridge multiple times, poking at the wall. Alex teased, "Bored yet?" She insisted she wasn't, but she clearly was itching for a screen fix. By evening, she flopped onto the couch, lamenting the "lack of anything to do," while Alex calmly insisted they hold out, reading quietly by the fireplace. Bella was unimpressed and hurled a pillow at him.

Day 2: Unfamiliar Freedoms

With no fresh input, Bella's mind started to wander. Memories of silly middle-school plays bubbled up, prompting them to write a parody "cabin experience" skit, complete with a bizarre character named "Sir Boredom." They spent hours riffing on silly lines, eventually performing a mini-show for each other, cracking up at its ridiculousness. Alex also found himself, with no texts or notifications, reflecting on a personal issue he'd been putting off. Somewhere in the emptiness, a new perspective formed. The day they'd dreaded as "stuck in the woods with nothing to do" became a creative spark.

Day 3: Comfort in Calm

By the final day, the pace slowed. They fished in the morning (without catching anything except random daydreams). Later, each read uninterrupted for hours, a luxury neither had allowed themselves in ages. Bella recalled, "I used to do this every weekend when I was 12. Why did I stop?" Alex's one-word answer: "Smartphones." By the end of the trip, Bella even left her phone on airplane mode for a while, savoring a sense of mental clarity. Sure, day-to-day life wouldn't always let them vanish to a cabin, but they discovered that sprinkling in small "boredom breaks" might be enough to glean the benefits.

Their story hints at what can happen when we step off the mental hamster wheel of constant input: we're more creative, more in tune with each other, and less frazzled.

Reevaluating "Nothing" as Something

One major barrier to letting ourselves be bored is the fear of "wasting time." But doing nothing is, in some sense, doing something. It's letting your mind roam, rest, or reflect. Think of farmland lying fallow to replenish nutrients. Our brains, awash in messages and headlines, rarely get that respite. Occasional empty space can be the mental equivalent of a recharge.

A corollary to this viewpoint is the concept of "JOMO", Joy of Missing Out (Turkle, 2015). It's a gentle rebellion against the default fear (FOMO) that we're missing big events or viral trends. JOMO suggests it's okay, even beneficial, to skip certain amusements or obligations in favor of quietly reconnecting with oneself. Boredom dovetails with this idea: choosing not to fill every gap with content. Let yourself meander. That might mean an idle Sunday afternoon where you resist the phone and see where your impulses lead you, maybe a walk, maybe painting an old shelf, maybe nothing at all. The point is that "nothingness" can open up mental and emotional space for deeper experiences to come through.

Enjoying Intentional Boredom Without Embracing

Chronic Boredom

Of course, not all boredom is blissful. Chronic boredom, where you feel perpetually unengaged, lacking direction, may signal deeper issues like depression, dissatisfaction with daily life, or a need for new challenges (Eastwood et al., 2012). The approach here isn't to remain bored forever but to cultivate short or moderate spells of idle time, letting your mind rest and roam. That might be five minutes on the couch with the phone on the other side of the room, or a half hour sitting in the yard without a playlist. The difference is that the boredom is chosen, not forced by circumstance.

Admittedly, if your job or lifestyle is already unfulfilling, adding more "nothingness" might not solve the real problem. But a dash of boredom can help clarify what changes you might want to make. If you're bored at work, you might realize how strongly you long to try a side project or develop a new skill. An intentionally bored mind can highlight desires or ideas you'd been ignoring in the daily rush.

Practical Ways to Embrace Boredom

Letting the Mind Wander

Start small. Set aside a few minutes each day to do absolutely nothing, no phone, no background music, no "productive" multi-tasking. Your mind might rebel at first, filling with anxious urges to check messages or do chores. If you gently resist, you may find yourself daydreaming, noticing new thoughts, or simply unwinding. You don't even have to track your breath as in formal meditation. Just be.

Doing Repetitive Tasks Without Distractions

Washing dishes by hand or folding laundry in silence can become a refreshing pocket of reflection. We're so used to layering a podcast or show on top of these chores but letting them unfold in quiet can be oddly soothing. Some ideas or memories might surface while you rinse plates or match socks.

Minimizing Mini-Fills

Those tiny moments, waiting in a café queue, sitting on the bus, even pausing at a red light, often get plugged with a quick phone check. We act as if 30 seconds of potential boredom is intolerable. Next time, try resisting. Look around. People-watch (discreetly). Maybe you'll strike up a thought about a new project, or you'll savor the atmosphere in a way you usually ignore. If you slip and grab your phone, notice that impulse with some amusement, and see if you can let it go next time.

Scheduling Unplanned Time

Our calendars bristle with events. Consider leaving a chunk, like an entire Sunday morning, completely open. No errands, no streaming backlog. You might find yourself so bored that you spontaneously start baking or tackling that half-abandoned craft. Or you might realize you haven't spoken to a certain friend for a while, prompting a heartfelt call. The point is to let boredom nudge you to purposeful action, rather than letting busyness or digital amusements soak up every hour.

The Brain's Need for Slack

Neuroscientists note that the brain thrives on "default mode network" time, moments when it isn't engaged in external tasks (Christoff et. al., 2011). This state is crucial for daydreaming, self-reflection, and memory consolidation. If we never allow mental slack, we risk impairing these functions. A short daily boredom break can feed your brain's need to drift, storing experiences, and allowing new patterns of insight to emerge.

Key Takeaways

- Boredom Is Becoming Endangered: Many of us have constant stimulation at our fingertips, leaving no room for idle moments. Research (Wilson et al., 2014) even shows some people prefer mild electric shocks to sitting quietly with no distractions.

- Idle Time Spurs Creativity: Letting the mind wander can lead to unexpected ideas and personal revelations (Elpidorou, 2014). Without occasional "fallow" mental fields, original insights might remain hidden.

- "Doing Nothing" Is Actually Doing Something: True boredom allows mental rest, reflection, or daydreaming. It can inspire more meaningful pursuits once the mind grows tired of being idle.

- Finding a Balanced Approach: Chronic boredom can signal deeper dissatisfaction, but short spells of chosen boredom can rejuvenate. Scheduling a bit of device-free emptiness might clarify your goals or spark new hobbies.

- Small Steps to Embrace Boredom: Simple acts like folding laundry with no podcast, taking a quiet walk, or leaving your phone aside for five minutes can gently reintroduce you to the fruitful stillness we often run from.

Boredom might seem like the enemy of modern life. Yet a close look reveals that short, deliberate periods of unoccupied time can be surprisingly beneficial. They let us rest, explore daydreams, and rediscover childlike creativity. Sure, the avalanche of apps and online shows is tempting, and it's fine to enjoy them. But sprinkling in some open space, like Alex and Bella did in their cabin experiment, can help you tune into deeper curiosities. Feeling "nothing to do" for a bit might unlock a realm of possibility, whether it's sketching a silly character, reflecting on a personal problem, or simply letting your mind roam free.

With this chapter, we near the end of our journey. In the upcoming, final chapter, we'll bring the threads together, reflecting on the overall lessons learned, how everything from "ignorance is bliss" to "fail spectacularly," from "humor in relationships" to "the lost art of boredom," can shape a more balanced, thoughtful life. Let's step forward with a renewed sense of calm, imagination, and maybe a dash of intentional emptiness, poised for the concluding insights ahead.

Chapter 13: Keep Laughing, Keep Growing

Perhaps growth is less about conquering every fear, and more about letting life's wonders and weirdness keep opening you

Long meanders through anxiety, dips into the cavern of depression, side quests into self-criticism, and glimpses of triumph in relationships or small daily joys have led to this concluding chapter. In some ways, these pages have spanned a personal odyssey, one in which fear gave way to resilience, heartbreak found a balm in humor, and self-discovery emerged among trials that once seemed endless. For all who have traveled these passages, there's an unmistakable sense that while this book ends, personal growth is an unfolding horizon, not a finish line.

Yet, here we are. Something about crossing a final threshold calls for reflection. The purpose is to gather what's been gleaned, a bit like pausing atop a hill to see the path behind and the plains ahead. Because after all the stories and coping strategies, the deeper hope is that these insights might continue resonating in subtle ways: a gentle shift in your morning routine, a more empathetic lens toward yourself and others, or a laughter-laced approach to a worry that arises.

Many have shaped this road: supportive people, fleeting strangers, the gentle nudge of professional help, or even chance encounters with a meaningful quote. In weaving together these themes, "ignorance is bliss" (sometimes), the value of perspective, ways to handle chaos, the gentle power of relationships, the art of failing better, the beauty of doing nothing. The abiding thread is humor and openness. These two qualities can lighten the journey and spark curiosity at every turn.

So, there are seven core principles I'd like to narrow down from all that we talked about.

Seven Core Principles for an Ongoing Adventure

1. Healing Rarely Follows a Straight Line

An image of self-improvement that is very familiar to many is one that makes a self-smooth, a clean, upward slope: start low, climb steadily, reach mastery. But reality tends to play out in a more serpentine trajectory. Two steps forward, one step back, a step sideways, maybe a jump forward, and a fall. Moments in which you feel invincible may be followed by unexpected slips into anxiety or self-doubt. This is normal.

Visualize progress less as a single shining ladder, more as a zigzagging trail that overall ascends. When you notice a backslide, it might be the brain needing rest, or old habits flaring up. It doesn't negate how far you've traveled; it just means there's another bend in the path. Over time, trust that each valley or plateau becomes part of a broader climb toward a more grounded, flexible sense of self (Neff, 2011). Understanding that these ups and downs are the norm can help soften the blow when they happen.

2. You're Stronger Than You Give Yourself Credit For

In earlier chapters, we saw how easily we label ourselves as fragile or behind, especially when mental health wavers. But if you pause to look honestly at your past, it may reveal remarkable resilience. Making it through heartbreak, panic attacks, financial worry, or just heavy daily stress requires real fortitude. Think of all the burdens you've carried so far. That track record is proof of your capacity, even if you sometimes feel powerless.

Each time you catch yourself thinking "I can't handle this," try recounting a time you overcame a smaller or similar struggle. This would remind you that fear can be loud but not always truthful. Resilience is the hidden undercurrent. Each day you find a way forward as a quiet power.

3. Don't Lose the Smile, Even When It's Hard

As the chapters unfolded, humor emerged as a sneaky, potent ally, from imagining anxious thoughts as frisky gremlins to introducing playful banter in relationships. Laughter is not about denying seriousness; it's about disarming the grip of dread or shame, turning a tidal wave into a manageable ripple. In darkness or panic, a slight smile or a quiet chuckle can reduce the panic monster.

This principle extends to daily mishaps. Coffee spills, awkward encounters, small humiliations. Observing these from a slightly amused vantage point can keep them from ballooning into catastrophes (Martin, 2018). Humor also bonds us with others. If we can share a lighthearted moment of life's oddities, we reaffirm our shared humanity. It's a gentle refusal to let negativity define the narrative. Some might see it as trivial, but a well-timed grin can tilt a situation from breakdown to breakthrough.

4. Growth Is a Lifelong, Iterative Process

Many of us fantasize about arriving at a definitive "I'm fixed now" moment, leading to discouragement when the more floating new fears arise, or familiar loops reappear. Growth is more cyclical. Life's every season has a way of illuminating the less-traveled corners of your psyche. New insecurities hanging out in the attic, or new depths to unearth in the basement. Instead of endless toil, think of it as an arc of a story: each chapter teaching you something along the way, changing your perspective, widening your empathy for others who are struggling.

One day, you might revisit these pages, discovering that a certain anecdote or method hits differently because your context changed. The repeated loop is not monotony; it's a spiral, hopefully moving upward with each pass. Embrace this cycle rather than yearning for a permanent "end." This attitude fosters gentleness toward yourself when confronting new problems or revisiting old ones.

5. Seek Out (and Build) a Supportive Community

Over the course of this book, relationships emerged as a critical factor. Whether it's the comedic relief that spouses share, the empathy a therapist provides, or the role of friends cheering your small steps. Humans thrive with connection. Even the most introverted or self-sufficient among us benefit from a friend's validating nod or a group that welcomes our quirks.

If certain relationships drain your energy or sow negativity, it's wise to reassess boundaries. The aim isn't to isolate yourself, but to lean into networks where you feel valued and safe. Meanwhile, you can pay that acceptance forward, learning to listen better, offering compassion rather than judgment, or simply showing up for a friend's small meltdown. Strong networks form from mutual presence. And in times of crisis, these bonds can be lifelines, reminding you that being seen and supported is a powerful antidote to life's darker currents (Brown, 2012).

6. Celebrate Every Incremental Victory

In a culture of bigger-better-faster, we often discount the small but essential victories: making it out of bed on a bleak day, pausing an anxious spiral before it escalates, or spending an extra moment on self-care. Noticing these small victories can keep you energized and increase the level of well-being. Seligman and Csikszentmihalyi (2000) explain how it makes sense to emphasize positive accomplishments, no matter how small, as it retrains the brain to pay attention to forward movement, and enables a upward spiral of confidence.

Some prefer a journal, jotting three micro-wins each evening. Others share them with a supportive friend. However, you choose, letting yourself feel that moment of "I did it!" fosters resilience. Think of it like feeding small logs to the campfire of your self-esteem, ensuring it stays lit against the night's chill. Each small flicker of success, over time, becomes a steady glow.

7. Pay It Forward Through Kindness

Climbing out of anxiety or depression, learning to channel humor, or finding self-compassion doesn't only help you; it can have an outward ripple effect. When you share a resource with a colleague who is struggling quietly, offer a tip from your own healing path, or gently reassure a friend that "they're not alone," you reinforce your own growth while giving them a lifeline. Raposa et al. (2016) note how providing support to others can boost one's own sense of empowerment and reduce stress responses.

There's a boomerang effect here. The empathy you cultivated under strain can become the warm hand someone else needs to hold. And in offering it, you remind yourself that your story, with all its scars, remains invaluable. Some call this the "wounded healer" archetype, where personal suffering becomes a well of compassion for the world. Whether you're passing on a therapy app link, volunteering at a helpline, or simply texting a friend "I'm here," each act of kindness cements the lessons you've learned and keeps the circle of human support turning.

What I mean is

Each principle above represents a strand of the tapestry we've woven through these chapters. And with them in mind, you stand at a threshold, this final page, holding the threads of your own narrative. There isn't a single grand flourish that answers all dilemmas, no final trick to guarantee perpetual contentment. But perhaps there's a fresh perspective: that being human is inherently a story of stumbling, learning, laughing, and stumbling again.

There might be days soon when you wake feeling unstoppable, forging ahead with zeal, using all the tactics and self-knowledge gleaned here. Then, unexpectedly, an anxious swirl or a wave of sadness might reappear. If so, remember that the dips don't erase the climb. Feeling wobbly isn't proof of failure, it's an echo that you're still in motion, still forging onward. In those moments, one of these seven ideas may resonate, or you might recall a snippet from earlier chapters about rethinking failure or discovering solace in a silly imaginative gesture.

No doubt you'll discover more lessons, possibly from volume two of this series (or from other books, mentors, or your own lived experiences). Everyone's adventure weaves through fresh territory over time. There's no pressing reason to rush. Along the way, rest in the knowledge that you carry enough resilience to greet new chapters with curiosity. Maybe there's even a small grin waiting, ready to lighten the load.

As you set this volume aside, see to how you might apply the unstructured calm of "boredom breaks," the balanced caution of "better safe than sorry," or the humorous approach to navigating heartbreak or panic. Instead of an explicit invitation or farewell, let these pages settle into your mind. If a quiet moment arises tonight or next week, you might find a stray insight drifting back to nudge you. A memory of a time you overcame adversity, or a whisper that laughter can shrink fear, or the recollection that heartbreak eventually eased into wisdom. You might just muse on how far you've traveled. And how many more roads await.

Thank you for reading, in the fullest sense. May your path continue with renewed humor, an open heart, and the gentle confidence that you're capable of ever-deepening growth. There's always another dawn, another perspective, another small triumph to savor. Keep going, keep laughing, and keep learning from the luminous, if sometimes bumpy, road of being fully human.

With love and optimism,

Felicity Hartwell

About the Author

Felicity Hartwell is a writer, a mental health advocate, and a champion of humor's healing powers, an experienced by experience survivor. The discovery of relatable storytelling and the transformative effect we have on each other through shared experience, leaving behind anxiety and depression, this is the journey she is taking us on, through them, alive, well, and thriving.

Felicity has used writing as her self-made therapy since the days when she filled cheap notebooks with doodles. Her singular style, often humorous and raw, tends to grab readers and leave them feeling less alone. Her warmth, homespun humor and down-to-earth wit shine as she translates big mental health concepts into personal anecdotes, and as running local support workshops ranging from journaling to "anxiety charades."

Felicity has had many professional faces over the years, but a constant through it all has been her desire to connect with people using words. She is drawn to the power of laughter as a force for disarming fear, and her instincts for how to make 'mental health speak' into relatable, real-life stories confirm it. If you can laugh at how ridiculous your fears are you rob them of their power, she believes, imbuing her readers with hope.

Felicity wrote this, as her first manuscript, Half Crazy, Fully Human, because she truly believed a book on mental wellness could also be thought-engaging and genuinely entertaining. She doesn't pull any punches on the hard stuff. Panic attacks in public places, the deaths of loved ones, the kind of self-loathing that all too often accompanies mental health issues. But she approaches it with compassion and playful mirth, like a friend you trust implicitly to hug you and tease you out of a sour mood. Even the pseudonym she chose, Felicity Hartwell, says it: Felicity is the happiness that is her goal, and Hartwell is a reminder of the heartfelt wellness at the heart of her message.

When she's not writing, Felicity hikes the scenic trails of her home state (a guaranteed antidote for anxiety, in her opinion), paints abstract watercolors that never quite stay within the lines, and devours self-help literature and stand-up comedy specials in equal parts, an odd pairing that she insists keeps her balanced. She is also the proud human of a rescue dog named Charlie, whose antics remind one to live in the moment.

Felicity now lives in the imaginary world of Flame Dance, a Northern State in Absurdistan, and writes, volunteers and speaks about mental health. She still sometimes talks to herself in funny voices, a childhood quirk turned self-soothing tool that she cheerfully advises anyone to try if they feel brave enough. Through her work, Felicity hopes readers feel seen, lifted, and reminded that being "half crazy" sometimes doesn't prevent you from being all-the-way, beautifully human.

References

Abagnale, F. W., & Redding, S. (2002). Catch me if you can: The true story of a real fake (First Broadway books movie tie-in edition). Broadway Books. http://catdir.loc.gov/catdir/samples/random045/00025063.html

American Psychiatric Association. (2020). Practice guideline for the treatment of patients with major depressive disorder(3rd ed.). APA Publishing.

Aronson, E., & Mills, J. (1959). The effect of severity of initiation on liking for a group. The Journal of Abnormal and Social Psychology, 59(2), 177–181. https://doi.org/10.1037/h0047195

Association for Psychological Science. (2024). Couples who laugh together, stay together – Association for Psychological Science – APS. Retrieved January 15, 2025, from https://www.psychologicalscience.org/news/utc-2024-feb-couples-who-laugh-together.html

Baikie, K. A., & Wilhelm, K. (2005). Emotional and physical health benefits of expressive writing. Advances in Psychiatric Treatment, 11(5), 338–346. https://doi.org/10.1192/apt.11.5.338

Baldwin, N. (1995). Edison: Inventing the century. University of Chicago Press. Retrieved March 10, 2025, from https://archive.org/details/edisoninventingc00bald

Beck, A. T. (1976a). Cognitive therapy and the emotional disorders. Meridian.

Beck, A. T. (1976b). Cognitive therapy and the emotional disorders. International Universities Press. https://ccl.on.worldcat.org/oclc/2330993

Beck, A. T., & Emery, G. (1985). Anxiety disorders and phobias: A cognitive perspective. Basic. http://archive.org/details/anxietydisorders00beck

Bertrand, M., & Mullainathan, S. (2004). Are Emily and Greg more employable than Lakisha and Jamal? A field experiment on labor market discrimination. American Economic Review, 94(4), 991–1013. https://doi.org/10.1257/0002828042002561

Brooks, R. (2009, May 15). Be cautious about first impressions: The case of Susan Boyle (and many others). Retrieved January 16, 2025, from https://www.drrobertbrooks.com/0905/

Brooks, S. K., Webster, R. K., Smith, L. E., Woodland, L., Wessely, S., & Rubin, G. J. (2020). The psychological impact of quarantine and how to reduce it: Rapid review of the evidence. The Lancet, 395(10227), 912–920. https://doi.org/10.1016/S0140-6736(20)30460-8

Burns, D. D. (with Internet Archive). (1989). The feeling good handbook. Plume Book. http://archive.org/details/feelinggoodhandbburn00burn

Butzer, B., & Kuiper, N. A. (2008). Humor use in romantic relationships: The effects of relationship satisfaction and pleasant versus conflict situations. The Journal of Psychology, 142(3), 245–260. https://doi.org/10.3200/JRLP.142.3.245-260

Casacalenda, N., Perry, J. C., & Looper, K. (2002). Remission in major depressive disorder: A comparison of pharmacotherapy, psychotherapy, and control conditions. American Journal of Psychiatry, 159(8), 1354–1360. https://doi.org/10.1176/appi.ajp.159.8.1354

Cheever, N. A., Rosen, L. D., Carrier, L. M., & Chavez, A. (2014). Out of sight is not out of mind: The impact of restricting wireless mobile device use on anxiety levels among low, moderate and high users. Computers in Human Behavior, 37, 290–297. https://doi.org/10.1016/j.chb.2014.05.002

Christoff, K., Gordon, A. M., & Smith, R. (2011). The role of spontaneous thought in human cognition. In R. Proctor & E. Capaldi (Eds.), Handbook of the psychology of science (pp. 255–268). Springer.

Diener, E., Oishi, S., & Tay, L. (2018). Advances in subjective well-being research. Nature Human Behaviour, 2(4), 253–260. https://doi.org/10.1038/s41562-018-0307-6

Dimidjian, S., Martell, C. R., & Herman-Dunn, R. (2014). Behavioral activation for depression. In D. H. Barlow (Ed.), Clinical handbook of psychological disorders (5th ed., pp. 353–393). Guilford Press. https://psycnet.apa.org/record/2014-05860-011

Duckworth, A. (2016). Grit: The power of passion and perseverance. Scribner. http://ebookcentral.proquest.com/lib/claremont/detail.action?docID=5685218

Dweck, C. S. (2006). Mindset: The new psychology of success (1st ed.). Random House. https://research.ebsco.com/linkprocessor/plink?id=43f6ccab-f3c5-38af-b30f-6be47038a3c9

Eastwood, J. D., Frischen, A., Fenske, M., & Smilek, D. (2012). The unengaged mind: Defining boredom in terms of attention. Perspectives on Psychological Science, 7(5), 482–495. https://doi.org/10.1177/1745691612456044

Edison, T. A. (1910). Thomas Alva Edison: Sixty years of an inventor's life (F. A. Jones, Ed.). John C. Winston. (Original anecdotes referenced in interviews and popular quotations.) https://www.loc.gov/item/08004377/

Edmonson, A. (1999). Psychological safety and learning behavior in work teams. Administrative Science Quarterly, 44(2), 350–383. https://doi.org/10.2307/2666999

Elpidorou, A. (2014). The bright side of boredom. Frontiers in Psychology, 5, 1245. https://doi.org/10.3389/fpsyg.2014.01245

Eskreis-Winkler, L., & Fishbach, A. (2019). Not learning from failure—the greatest failure of all. Psychological Science, 30(12), 1733–1744. https://doi.org/10.1177/0956797619881133

Food and Drug Administration (FDA). (2024). Overview of our role regulating and approving drugs | Video series. Retrieved January 17, 2025, from https://www.fda.gov/drugs/information-consumers-and-patients-drugs/overview-our-role-regulating-and-approving-drugs-video-series

Fredrickson, B. L. (2001). The role of positive emotions in positive psychology: The broaden-and-build theory of positive emotions. American Psychologist, 56(3), 218–226. https://doi.org/10.1037/0003-066X.56.3.218

Gilovich, T., & Medvec, V. H. (1995). The experience of regret: What, when, and why. Psychological Review, 102(2), 379–395. https://doi.org/10.1037/0033-295X.102.2.379

Goldin, C., & Rouse, C. (2000). Orchestrating impartiality: The impact of "blind" auditions on female musicians. American Economic Review, 90(4), 715–741. https://doi.org/10.1257/aer.90.4.715

Gottman, J., & Silver, N. (2012). What makes love last? How to build trust and avoid betrayal. Simon & Schuster. https://www.google.com/books/edition/What_Makes_Love_Last/TOzCA3ZnvT8C?hl=en&gbpv=1&printsec=frontcover

Grant, G. (Director). (1555537136). Bouncing back from rejection [Video recording]. Retrieved March 12, 2025, from https://www.ted.com/talks/worklife_with_adam_grant_bouncing_back_from_rejection

Gray, P. (2013). Free to learn: Why unleashing the instinct to play will make our children happier, more self-reliant, and better students for life. Basic Books. https://www.google.com/books/edition/Free_to_Learn/2IgkAIMG3qgC?hl=en&gbpv=1&dq=Why+unleashing+the+instinct+to+play+will+make+our+children+happier,+more+self-reliant,+and+better+students+for+life&printsec=frontcover

Hammen, C. (2018). Risk factors for depression: An autobiographical review. Annual Review of Clinical Psychology, 14, 1–15. https://doi.org/10.1146/annurev-clinpsy-050817-084811

Haselton, M. G., & Buss, D. M. (2000). Error management theory: A new perspective on biases in cross-sex mind reading. Journal of Personality and Social Psychology, 78(1), 81–91. https://doi.org/10.1037/0022-3514.78.1.81

Holmes, J., & Marra, M. (2002). Having a laugh at work: How humor contributes to workplace culture. Journal of Pragmatics, 34(12), 1683–1710. https://doi.org/10.1016/S0378-2166(02)00032-2

ICAO (International Civil Aviation Organization). (2019). Safety management manual (4th ed.). Retrieved January 18, 2025, from https://www.icao.int/safety/SafetyManagement/Documents/SMM%204th%20edition%20highlights.pdf

Inagaki, T. K., & Eisenberger, N. I. (2016). Giving support to others reduces sympathetic nervous system–related responses to stress. Psychophysiology, 53(4), 427–435. https://doi.org/10.1111/psyp.12578

Inzlicht, M., Shenhav, A., & Olivola, C. Y. (2018). The effort paradox: Effort is both costly and valued. Trends in Cognitive Sciences, 22(4), 337–349. https://doi.org/10.1016/j.tics.2018.01.007

Jacobson, N. S., Martell, C. R., & Dimidjian, S. (2001). Behavioral activation treatment for depression: Returning to contextual roots. Clinical Psychology: Science and Practice, 8(3), 255–270. https://doi.org/10.1093/clipsy.8.3.255

Kabat-Zinn, J. (1990). Full catastrophe living: Using the wisdom of your body and mind to face stress, pain, and illness.Dell.

Kahneman, D., & Deaton, A. (2010). High income improves evaluation of life but not emotional well-being. Proceedings of the National Academy of

Sciences, 107(38), 16489–
16493. https://doi.org/10.1073/pnas.1011492107

Killingsworth, M. A., Kahneman, D., & Mellers, B. (2023).
Income and emotional well-being: A conflict
resolved. Proceedings of the National Academy of
Sciences, 120(10),
e2208661120. https://doi.org/10.1073/pnas.2208661120

Kross, E., & Ayduk, O. (2011). Making meaning out of
negative experiences by self-distancing. Current
Directions in Psychological Science, 20(3), 187–
191. https://doi.org/10.1177/0963721411408883

Kurtz, L. E., & Algoe, S. B. (2015). Putting laughter in context:
Shared laughter as behavioral indicator of relationship
well-being. Personal Relationships, 22(4), 573–
590. https://doi.org/10.1111/pere.12095

Lawson, A. (1978). Social Origins of Depression. By George
Brown and Tirril Harris. (Pp. 399; illustrated; £12.50.)
Tavistock: London. 1978. Psychological Medicine, 8(4),
717–720. https://doi.org/10.1017/S0033291700018924

Lucas, H. C., & Goh, J. M. (2009). Disruptive technology: How
Kodak missed the digital photography revolution. The
Journal of Strategic Information Systems, 18(1), 46–
55. https://doi.org/10.1016/j.jsis.2009.01.002

Ma Bloomfield, S. F., Stanwell-Smith, R., Crevel, R. W. R., &
Pickup, J. (2006). Too clean, or not too clean: The
hygiene hypothesis and home hygiene. Clinical &
Experimental Allergy, 36(4), 402–
425. https://doi.org/10.1111/j.1365-2222.2006.02463.x

Martin, R. A., & Ford, T. (2018). The psychology of humor: An
integrative approach. Elsevier Science &

Technology. http://ebookcentral.proquest.com/lib/clare mont/detail.action?docID=5457186

Maslach, C., Schaufeli, W. B., & Leiter, M. P. (2001). Job burnout. Annual Review of Psychology, 52(1), 397–422. https://doi.org/10.1146/annurev.psych.52.1.397

Mayo Clinic. (2023). Stress relief from laughter? It's no joke. Retrieved January 19, 2025, from https://www.mayoclinic.org/healthy-lifestyle/stress-management/in-depth/stress-relief/art-20044456

McPherson, M., Smith-Lovin, L., & Cook, J. M. (2001). Birds of a feather: Homophily in social networks. Annual Review of Sociology, 27, 415–444. https://doi.org/10.1146/annurev.soc.27.1.415

Medical News Today. (2023, January 11). How journaling can help you manage anxiety and stress. Retrieved January 20, 2025, from https://www.medicalnewstoday.com/articles/ journaling-for-anxiety

Meichenbaum, D. (1985). Stress inoculation training. Pergamon Press. https://melissainstitute.org/wp-content/uploads/2015/10/Stress_Inoculation_052806.pdf

Meinchenbaum, D. H., & Deffenbacher, J. L. (1988). Stress inoculation training. https://doi.org/10.1177/0011000088161005

Mednick, S. C., Ehrman, M., & OverDrive, I. (2013). Take a nap! Change your life (Vol. 1–1 online resource: illustrations). Workman Publishing. http://link.overdrive.com/?websiteID=262&titleID=1224585

Neff, K. (2011). Self-compassion: The proven power of being kind to yourself (First William Morrow paperback edition). William Morrow. https://debphelps.com/wp-content/uploads/2018/09/Self-Compassion_-The-Proven-Pow-Kristin-Neff.pdf

NIMH (National Institute of Mental Health). (2018). Depression basics. Retrieved January 21, 2025, from https://www.nimh.nih.gov/health/publications/depression

Norton, M. I., Mochon, D., & Ariely, D. (2012). The IKEA effect: When labor leads to love. Journal of Consumer Psychology, 22(3), 453–460. https://doi.org/10.1016/j.jcps.2011.08.002

Page, S. E. (2008, August 31). The difference | Princeton University Press. Retrieved January 22, 2025, from https://press.princeton.edu/books/paperback/9780691138541/the-difference

Parker, G., Roy, K., & Eyers, K. (2003). Cognitive behavior therapy for depression? Choose horses for courses. American Journal of Psychiatry, 160(5), 825–834. https://doi.org/10.1176/appi.ajp.160.5.825

Pew Research Center. (2015). The demographics of social media users. Retrieved January 23, 2025, from https://www.pewresearch.org/internet/

Plomin, R., DeFries, J. C., Knopik, V. S., & Neiderhiser, J. M. (2016). Top 10 replicated findings from behavioral genetics. Perspectives on Psychological Science, 11(1), 3–23. https://doi.org/10.1177/1745691615617439

Reuters/Ipsos. (2013, August). Social situation in many communities [Poll statistics]. Retrieved January 24, 2025, from the Reuters/Ipsos polling archives.

Ringelmann, M. (1913). Recherches sur les moteurs animés: Travail de l'homme [Research on animate sources of power: Work of man]. Annales de l'Institut National Agronomique, 2(12), 1–40.

Russell, J., & Blowers, A. (2013). Risk, vulnerability, and nuclear energy: The perils of "better safe than sorry." Society & Natural Resources, 26(8), 846–859. https://doi.org/10.1080/08941920.2013.785115

Schmitt, M. H., Stears, K., & Shrader, A. M. (2015). Zebras as possible "watchdogs" for wildebeests, how grouping dynamics influence vigilance. Applied Animal Behaviour Science, 169, 31–35. https://doi.org/10.1016/j.applanim.2015.05.011

Schore, A. N. (2019). Right brain psychotherapy (pp. xii, 356). W. W. Norton & Company. https://psycnet.apa.org/record/2019-12810-000

Schoenfeld, B. J. (2010). The mechanisms of muscle hypertrophy and their application to resistance training. Journal of Strength and Conditioning Research, 24(10), 2857–2872. https://doi.org/10.1519/JSC.0b013e3181e840f3

Seligman, M. E. P., & Csikszentmihalyi, M. (2000). Positive psychology: An introduction. American Psychologist, 55(1), 5–14. https://doi.org/10.1037/0003-066X.55.1.5

Seligman, M. E. P., Steen, T. A., Park, N., & Peterson, C. (2005). Positive Psychology Progress: Empirical Validation of Interventions. American Psychologist,

60(5), 410–421. https://doi.org/10.1037/0003-066X.60.5.410

Sweeny, K., Melnyk, D., Miller, W., & Shepperd, J. A. (2010). Information avoidance: Who, what, when, and why. Review of General Psychology, 14(4), 340–353. https://doi.org/10.1037/a0021288

Thompson, D. C., Rivara, F. P., & Thompson, R. (2018). Helmets for preventing head and facial injuries in bicyclists. Cochrane Database of Systematic Reviews, (1). https://doi.org/10.1002/14651858.CD001855.pub5

Thondike, E. L. (1920). A constant error in psychological ratings. Journal of Applied Psychology, 4(1), 25–29. https://doi.org/10.1037/h0071663

Todorov, A., Mandisodza, A. N., Goren, A., & Hall, C. C. (2005). Inferences of competence from faces predict election outcomes. Science, 308(5728), 1623–1626. https://doi.org/10.1126/science.1110589

Turkle, S. (2015). Reclaiming conversation: The power of talk in a digital age. Penguin Press.

Tusser, T. (1562). A hundreth good pointes of husbandrie. London: Richard Tottel. (Original work published 1557.)

University of Birmingham commentary (as cited in Kanazawa & Li, 2018). [Placeholder—no direct link or date provided.] Retrieved January 25, 2025, from internal references.

Van Zalk, M. H. W., Kerr, M., Branje, S. J., Stattin, H., & Meeus, W. H. J. (2010). Peer contagion and adolescent depression. Development and Psychopathology, 22(1), 87–98. https://doi.org/10.1017/S0954579409990265

Vygotsky, L. S. (1978). Mind in society: The development of higher psychological processes. Harvard University Press.

Waldinger, R. (2016). What makes a good life? Lessons from the longest study on happiness [Video]. TED Conferences. https://www.ted.com/talks/robert_walding er_what_makes_a_good_life_lessons_from_the_longe st_study_on_happiness

Wang, D., Song, C., & Barabási, A.-L. (2013). Quantifying long-term scientific impact. Science, 342(6154), 127–132. https://doi.org/10.1126/science.1237825

Wilson, T. D., Reinhard, D. A., Westgate, E. C., Gilbert, D. T., Ellerbeck, N., Hahn, C., Brown, C., & Shaked, A. (2014). Just think: The challenges of the disengaged mind. Science, 345(6192), 75–77. https://doi.org/10.1126/science.1250830

Wu, T. (2016). The attention merchants: The epic scramble to get inside our heads. Faculty Books. https://scholarship.law.columbia.edu/books/64

Yerkes, R. M., & Dodson, J. D. (1908). The relation of strength of stimulus to rapidity of habit-formation. Journal of Comparative Neurology and Psychology, 18(5), 459–482. https://doi.org/10.1002/cne.920180503

Ziv, A. (2010). The Social Function of Humor in Interpersonal Relationships. Society, 47(1), 11–18. https://doi.org/10.1007/s12115-009-9283-9

www.ingramcontent.com/pod-product-compliance
Lightning Source LLC
Chambersburg PA
CBHW031212270326
41931CB00006B/537